DISCARD

COLOR ATLAS
of
DOMESTIC VIOLENCE

COLOR ATLAS
of
DOMESTIC
VIOLENCE

S. SCOTT POLSKY, MD, FACEP
Medical Director of Emergency Services
Lafayette General Medical Center
Lafayette, Louisiana

Associate Professor
Clinical Emergency Medicine
Northeastern Ohio Universities
College of Medicine
Rootstown, Ohio

JENIFER MARKOWITZ, ND, RNC, WHNP
Coordinator of Victim Services
The DOVE Program
Summa Health System
Akron, Ohio

With 208 illustrations

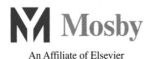

An Affiliate of Elsevier

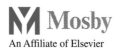

An Affiliate of Elsevier

11830 Westline Industrial Drive
St. Louis, Missouri 63146

Color Atlas of Domestic Violence
Copyright © 2004, Mosby, Inc. All rights reserved.

ISBN 0-323-01714-2

NOTICE

Medicine is an ever-changing field. Standard safety precautions must be followed, but as new research and
clinical experience broaden our knowledge, changes in treatment and drug therapy may become necessary
or appropriate. Readers are advised to check the most current product information provided by the manu-
facturer of each drug to be administered to verify the recommended dose, the method and duration of
administration, and contraindications. It is the responsibility of the licensed prescriber, relying on experience and knowledge of the patient, to determine dosages and the best treatment for each individual patient.
Neither the publisher nor the authors assume any liability for any injury and/or damage to persons or property arising from this publication.

International Standard Book Number 0-323-01714-2

Executive Editor: Susan R. Epstein
Developmental Editor: Robyn L. Brinks
Publishing Services Manager: John Rogers
Senior Project Managers: Beth Hayes, Kathleen L. Teal
Senior Designer: Kathi Gosche

Printed in the United States of America

Last digit is the print number: 9   8   7   6   5   4   3   2   1

For
Jill Bunnell and Teresa Roe
who continue to raise the standard of care
for victims of violence.

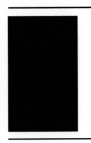

PHOTOGRAPH EDITOR

David Effron, MD, FACEP
Assistant Professor
Case Western Reserve University
Department of Emergency Medicine
MetroHealth Medical Center
Emergency Medicine Consultant
Cleveland Clinic Foundation
Cleveland, Ohio

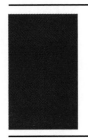

CONTRIBUTORS

Eileen F. Baker, MD
Emergency Medical Services Medical
    Director
Union Hospital
Dover, Ohio

James Connors, DMD, MD
Chief Resident
Department of Oral and Maxillofacial
    Surgery
Case Western Reserve University
University Hospitals
Cleveland, Ohio

David Effron, MD, FACEP
Assistant Professor
Case Western University
Department of Emergency Medicine
MetroHealth Medical Center
Emergency Medicine Consultant
Cleveland Clinic Foundation
Cleveland, Ohio

Lisa J. Kohler, MD
Chief Medical Examiner
Summit County Medical Examiner's Office
Akron, Ohio

Justin Lavin, Jr., MD, FACOG
Associate Chair and Associate Program
    Director
Department of Obstetrics and Gynecology
Akron General Medical Center
Akron, Ohio
Chief, Maternal-Fetal Medicine
Summa Health System
Akron, Ohio
Professor
Department of Obstetrics and Gynecology
N.E.O.U.C.O.M.
Rootstown, Ohio

Douglas J. Lowery, MS, MD
Chief Resident Orthopaedic Surgery
Summa Orthopaedics
Akron, Ohio

Lori Sieboldt Lowery, MS, MD
Emergency Medicine Staff Physician
Emergency Medicine Physicians, Inc.
Parma Community General Hospital
Parma, Ohio

Alan Markowitz, MD
Co-Chief
Cardiothoracic Surgery
University Hospitals of Cleveland
Case Western Reserve University
Cleveland, Ohio

Michael Powers, DDS, MS
Associate Professor and Chair
Department of Oral and Maxillofacial
    Surgery
School of Dentistry
Case Western Reserve University
Cleveland, Ohio
Chief, Division of Oral and Maxillofacial
    Surgery
Department of Surgery
Rainbow Babies' and Children's Hospitals
University Hospitals of Cleveland
Cleveland, Ohio

**Valorie K. Prulhiere, RN, BSN, FNE,
    SANE-A**
Forensic Nurse Examiner
The DOVE Program, Summa Health System
Akron, Ohio

Paula Renker, PhD, RNc
Assistant Professor
College of Nursing
University of Akron
Akron, Ohio

Scott D. Weiner, MD
Director, Orthopaedic Resident Education
Summa Health System
Associate Professor, Orthopaedic Surgery
Northeastern Ohio Universities College of
    Medicine
Akron, Ohio

REVIEWERS

Sue Hagedorn, RN, PhD, PNP
Associate Professor
University of Colorado Health Sciences
    Center
Denver, Colorado

**Georgia A. Pasqualone, MSN, MSFS,
    RN, DABFN**
Clinical Nurse Specialist/Forensic Nurse
    Consultant
Staff Development/Emergency Department
Winchester Hospital
Winchester, Massachusetts

Kelly A. Robinson, MD, FAAEM
Medical Director of Emergency Services
Aurora Lakeland Medical Center
Elkhorn, Wisconsin

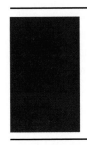

PREFACE

The *Color Atlas of Domestic Violence* provides an illustrative overview of domestic violence–related injury. It is meant as a tool for clinicians, regardless of specialty, because domestic violence–related complaints may be screened for and observed across the health care continuum. The ultimate goal of the *Color Atlas of Domestic Violence* is to increase the index of suspicion for all professionals involved in patient care. The authors hope clinicians will also examine hospital and practice protocols regarding screening, assessment, and referrals for victims of domestic violence, with an eye toward safety, universality, and collaboration.

A brief note about terminology: although *intimate partner violence* is the term more frequently used for domestic violence today by those working closely with the issue, the term *domestic violence* is still more recognizable to the majority of clinicians, as well as attorneys and law enforcement personnel, who will also find this text a valuable resource. Because of this, *domestic violence* is predominantly used throughout the body of the text.

The photographs in this book were taken from a variety of clinical arenas, including the emergency departments of several Level I trauma centers, a forensic nurse examiner program, and county medical examiner's offices. The vast majority of the photographs are 35 mm, although digital photography was used, as well. Although 35-mm film provides the sharpest images with the truest color, digital photography is being utilized in increasing frequency, and it was deemed important to have these types of images represented. Many clinicians utilize digital photography for documenting wound progression, skin conditions, and other clinical presentations. Documentation of intentional injury can be added to the list of reasons to keep *any* type of camera available in the health care setting.

The references and resources in this book were chosen in part because of the broad range of disciplines represented in the literature. Domestic violence is not *owned* by any particular specialty, and this is evidenced by the position statements of a variety of professional health care organizations and in the clinical research conducted by nursing, clinical medicine, forensic pathology, and others. With the advent and entrenchment of the Internet, there is also a wide range of on-line sites dedicated to domestic violence and the special needs of different populations around the globe: gay, lesbian, bisexual, and transgendered (GLBT) victims and their families; clergy working with violence in synagogues, churches, and mosques; migrant farmworkers; refugees; the disabled; and adolescents coping with dating violence. The list is seemingly endless. Quality sites and recommended resources were included in the book. They are not, however, the definitive list. Clinicians should explore the available resources on the Internet and elsewhere and make time to familiarize themselves with those serving their own communities.

Chapter 1 of the *Atlas* examines the clinician approach to domestic violence in the health care setting. This includes a brief review of the epidemiology and physical and emotional sequelae of domestic violence. Screening for domestic violence is described, including a review of barriers to and protocols for screening. This chapter also examines clinical clues, the process for documentation of injury, and referring patients safely and appropriately.

Chapter 2 begins the photographic portion of the *Atlas,* describing injury patterns and patterned injury in the domestic violence patient. Descriptors for injury are reviewed, as are types of injury seen as a result of particular types of blunt force trauma.

Chapter 3 examines the clinical approach to patients with serious or multiple trauma. The forensic approach to the patient is described, including techniques for collecting and preserving evidence and photographing injuries. The primary and secondary survey of trauma patients is also reviewed in this chapter.

Chapter 4 is an in-depth look at penetrating injuries. This chapter is meant to serve as an introduction to firearms and ballistics information for clinicians who may not have prior exposure to this topic. The strong association between firearms and lethality in the violent relationship makes the issue of penetrating trauma particularly compelling. Sharp force injuries are also reviewed in this chapter.

Chapters 5 through 10 address injury to specific areas of the body, including injury to the pregnant abdomen (Chapter 8). These chapters serve as a comprehensive illustration of the scope and breadth of domestic violence–related injuries. Radiographic images are incorporated with wound photographs throughout this section of the book. The chapters carefully examine situations that may be addressed in the course of routine visits; signs and symptoms of emergency conditions are explicitly outlined, including appropriateness of specialty referrals. As a component of the chapter on genital injury (Chapter 9), the issue of sexual violence is also explicitly addressed.

Chapter 11 looks specifically at special considerations for patients coping with domestic violence. The chapter briefly reviews issues related to same-sex violence, violence against persons with disabilities, violence against the elderly, culture and abuse, and children who witness violence. The chapter serves as an introduction to these issues and provides detailed resources for the clinician looking for additional information on any one of these topics. Suggested websites, videos, articles, and books are provided as a part of the reference list.

ACKNOWLEDGMENTS

Summa Health System, and in particular, The DOVE Program, supported this project and for that we are especially appreciative. Special thanks to the following people who provided the intangibles that made this book a reality: Colleen O'Brien, RN; Meghan Garland, RN, CNM; Elizabeth Madigan, PhD, RN; Mary Hancock, MD; Sheila Steer, MD; Lisa Kohler, MD; Thomas Marshall, DDS; Linda Breedlove, RN, MBA; Detective Bertina King; Rockie Brockway; James Flynn; and of course, our families.

S. Scott Polsky, MD, FACEP
Jenifer Markowitz, ND, RNc, WHNP

Contents

COLOR ATLAS
of
DOMESTIC
VIOLENCE

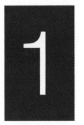

Clinician's Approach to Domestic Violence

Jenifer Markowitz • S. Scott Polsky • Paula Renker

EPIDEMIOLOGY

Intimate partner violence (IPV) is one of the biggest public health issues facing health care providers today. In 1998 an estimated 1 million incidents of IPV occurred in the United States, 85% of which were targeted toward women.[1] Although IPV occurs to both men and women, women make up the overwhelming majority of victims and available statistics underscore this fact. In 1998 women were the victims in 72% of murders committed by an intimate partner and were the victims in 85% of nonlethal partner violence.[1] In the National Violence Against Women Survey, 22% of surveyed women reported a history of IPV compared with 7% of men surveyed. Women were more likely to be injured during an incidence of IPV than men were—39% versus 25%, respectively. In general, 64% of women who reported a history of violent victimization after age 18 were victimized by an intimate partner.[2] Of additional concern is the prevalence of physical abuse during pregnancy. Research on abuse in pregnancy, including women over and under the age of 20, identified rates ranging from 5.2% to 36%.[3-9]

While the statistics above reflect the prevalence of physical abuse, the terms violence and abuse against women also represent sexual violence and psychological or emotional battering, including threats of physical and sexual assault. These three components were identified as being essential for defining the scope of violence against women by a panel of experts organized by the Centers for Disease Control (CDC) from government, private sector, and educational/research arenas.[10] Definitions and associated prevalence for each of the violence components proposed by the CDC panel and others are as follows:

- Physical abuse or violence: "The intentional use of physical force with the potential for causing death, disability, injury, or harm" (p. 11).[11]
- Sexual violence or abuse: "Use of physical force (and intimidation and pressure) to compel a person to engage in a sexual act against her or his will, whether or not the act is completed" (p. 12).[11] The magnitude of the problem of intimate partner sexual abuse is revealed in the associated prevalence rates. Approximately 1.5 million of the 2.1 million women who are raped each year in the United States are raped by their intimate

1

partners.[2] Plichta and Falik[12] used survey data from a sample of 1821 nonpregnant women from the Commonwealth Fund 1998 Survey of Women's Health to identify life-time sexual violence experiences from intimate and nonintimate partners. Intimate part-ner lifetime sexual violence, which included childhood sexual incest, was identified by 18.5% of the women, while 4.4% of the women had experienced sexual, nonintimate violence.

- Emotional or psychological abuse is defined as ". . . involving (emotional) trauma to the victim caused by acts, or coercive tactics" (p. 62).[11] Quantifying prevalence of emotional abuse is difficult because there are many different definitions of abuse used in research studies. Prevalence rates of emotional abuse range from a low of 5.9% to a high of 44%, with the low and high values representing emotional abuse during pregnancy.[3,8,9,13-17] Some researchers and policy makers may only consider emotional abuse as an act of vio-lence when it is associated with acts of physical or sexual assault. Emotional abuse as defined by women includes threats of violence, suicide, or abandonment; threats to chil-dren; blackmail; restricting access to friends and family; controlling money; and endless blaming, denigrating, and cursing.[18,19]

PHYSICAL AND EMOTIONAL SEQUELAE TO ABUSE

While the acute ramifications of physical abuse are graphically presented in this text, it is important to remember that abuse affects both body and spirit. Emotional or psychological consequences of violence occur in addition to the trauma caused by physical and sexual abuse. The sequelae of emotional abuse that often covary with past or current physical pregnancy abuse, include depression, diminished self-esteem, disassociative disorders, and post-traumatic stress disorder.[20-22] Women have described verbal and psychological abuse including coercion, isolation, deprivation, threats, humiliation, and emotional distance as, or more, detrimental than physical abuse.[16,21,23,24] Although physical aggression may be isolated and episodic, the psychological burden of emotional abuse and battering is ongoing, lasting beyond the physi-cal bruises and bleeding and may include fears of future trauma.[25,26,27]

The serious implications of the prevalence of sexual abuse are intensified by the associated physical and psychologic complications including poorer mental health (depression and anxiety) and physical health (disabilities, chronic conditions, and lower self-esteem), as well as dimin-ished access to health care.[12,28] Physical consequences of sexual assault include unwanted preg-nancy, sexually transmitted diseases, low birth-weight infants, and requests for abortion.[29-31]

Abuse during pregnancy exemplifies the dangerous interplay between physical, sexual, and emotional abuse with both short- and long-term direct and indirect effects on the mother and developing fetus.[16,17,32] Abused women are more likely to experience miscarriages and abor-tions, increased substance use, inadequate prenatal care, lower pregnancy weight gain, trauma, and postpartum depression.[31,33-36] In addition, their infants are more likely to be of low birth weight or have lower birth weights than infants of mothers who are not abused.[33,35-37]

Although the chronic effects of physical and sexual abuse are often devastating, an even more drastic and final consequence of abuse is homicide. Homicides at the hands of intimate partners have decreased by 69% since 1976, with actual numbers more pronounced for male victims than for female victims. Between 1976 and 1999, approximately 11% of homicides were committed by an intimate partner. However, women are still more likely to be killed by an intimate partner than men are, and this number remains consistently higher for every age-group. Firearms were responsible for most deaths caused by an intimate partner, although the number of deaths by firearms saw the sharpest decrease during this time period compared with homicides committed with other weapons.[1]

ASSESSING AND INTERVENING IN DOMESTIC VIOLENCE

Many victims of IPV never explicitly disclose the violence in their homes. However, they do access health care resources, often repeatedly, for treatment of injuries and stress-related illnesses. Of women injured by an intimate, 30% sought medical treatment for direct injuries.[2] The Commonwealth Fund conducted a survey of women that included questions about violence and health care. Of women who reported a history of abuse, 21% rated their health as fair or poor and identified a disability or illness that prevented them from working. Abused women who experience depression and anxiety often approach health care workers for mental health assessment and intervention. Regardless of illness, however, women who had been victimized had difficulty accessing health care services, including obtaining prescriptions and being seen by specialists. This also included mental health services—14% of women who had been victimized reported not being able to access a mental health professional compared with just 5% of women with no abuse history.

VIOLENCE SCREENING

Universal screening (or assessment) for domestic violence has been promoted as an integral component of prenatal and primary care by many national health organizations.[38-41] The goals of violence screening or assessment are to end the patient's isolation, make connections, and to review options.[42] This process will optimally result in the victims of abuse becoming sufficiently empowered to make safe and healthy choices for themselves and their children. Although universal screening has been widely promoted, many health care providers do not include it in their standard protocols.[7,43-46] Rates of screening for domestic violence differ according to the specialty of the health care provider. Physicians in primary care settings, including managed care or health maintenance organizations, have reported screening rates ranging from 1.5% to 26%.[47-50] Prevalence of screening estimates by obstetricians and gynecologists range from 10% to 30%.[38,43,44,49,51]

Domestic violence is often overlooked and undertreated in the emergency and trauma setting. Women make an estimated 547,000 visits annually to the emergency department for treatment of injuries from assault.[52] However, in a survey of Michigan shelters, half of the battered women and their advocates reported negative experiences in the emergency department including feeling humiliation and blame, not being identified as battered women, having their abuse minimized, and being given insufficient referrals.[53] This is problematic in light of the fact that approximately 22% to 27% of women presenting to an emergency department have been the victims of physical or nonphysical domestic violence in the prior year.[55-58] Feldhaus and associates[56] reported that 7.2% of emergency department visits were because of acute battering injuries and 11.5% were from stress from partner abuse. A study of six Pennsylvania and five California community emergency departments found that 2.2% of women had acute trauma from abuse, 14.4% had been physically or sexually abused in the past, and 36.9% had been physically or emotionally abused sometime in their lives.[57] Moreover, the sensitivity of the trauma registry in documenting violence against women is only 57% effective.[59] Clearly there is room for improvement.

BARRIERS TO SCREENING AND ACKNOWLEDGMENT OF ABUSE

There are a number of barriers to clinician involvement in domestic violence. Social issues include a societal tolerance of violence, desensitization through exposure, implicit and explicit social norms, and power inequities in relationships. Involvement is also limited by personal factors. These include gender bias and a personal history of abuse. Some health care workers have idealized concepts of family life that interfere with their judgment. Privacy concerns and a sense of powerlessness can also interfere with involvement. Professional factors such as time constraints and inadequate skills will negatively affect domestic violence screening. A professional relationship with the abuser may cause the health care worker to avoid asking the necessary questions. Professional detachment may also create a barrier between the health care provider and the domestic violence victim that inhibits discovery. There are also institutional and legal factors that decrease domestic violence screening. Many professionals fear legal involvement in the form of lengthy depositions or court appearances. Often, institutional resources are limited and policies are inadequate or unclear.[60]

In addition to barriers to screening identified by health care professionals, several barriers have been identified that can affect women's willingness to acknowledge abuse when asked. These barriers fall under the general organizing categories of personal, health care, and legal areas. Women relate that they are afraid that if they acknowledge they are abused and the partner finds out there will be reprisals from their partner.[47,61,62] Women experiencing domestic violence state that they are concerned the police will become involved and their partner might be incarcerated if they acknowledge abuse in their relationship. They also have concerns their children might be taken from them and given to the perpetrator's family or placed in foster care if the authorities find out about the abuse.[33,45,62-66] Abused women relate that shame and embarrassment keep them from acknowledging abuse.[62,65,67] Although these barriers may keep women from independently identifying they are abused, many state they would acknowledge the abuse if they were asked directly.[54,61,62,68] Women experiencing domestic violence also identified system-related barriers including the fact that physicians are "too busy."[47,50,69] Health care providers are often perceived as uncaring because they do not understand the consequences of domestic violence and appear to ridicule or isolate women who acknowledge domestic violence but refuse to file a report to the police.[67,69,70]

Before health care providers can accurately assess potential victims of IPV, they must first understand the cycle of violence, which consists of three phases or stages (Box 1-1). Frank and Rodowski[20] describe the cycle of violence as including both abusive and gratifying aspects that oscillate in a somewhat predictable fashion. They state that abuse often begins with a close, mutual relationship that becomes increasingly exclusive, allowing the perpetrator to isolate the victim from her friends and family. Violence appears slowly and insidiously or suddenly, but generally there is a "testing" mode with shoving or a pushing that escalates into more serious tactics. If the victim has sufficient support to stand up to the assailant to say that physical assault, in any form, is unacceptable, the violence can sometimes be eliminated. However, if the limitations are not accepted, physical and emotional assaults often intensify. After an abusive episode, the abuser frequently appears contrite, cooperative, and remorseful. The abuser may even return to "courting behavior" in which he is seductive and openly loving. Although victims develop insight into the two modes of behavior, they often cling to the hope that the partner will change and that their relationship can continue.

Health care providers must also understand why victims feel unable to leave an abusive relationship. A victim's reluctance to comply with the clinician's opinion of the best course of action should not be seen as a sign of apathy or unwillingness to recognize a complex and difficult situation. Extracting oneself from an abusive relationship cannot be accomplished on another person's timeline or to another person's specifications. See Box 1-2 for a list of some of the reasons victims stay in battering relationships. Coker and others[71] describe the psychological vulnerability that women often experience in an abusive relationship as an intense vulnerability or susceptibility to danger (physical and/or emotional), as well as a feeling of disempowerment and loss of control in their relationship with their partner. Other concerns that are frequently cited by victims of abuse that keep them from leaving are identified in Box 1-2.

Box 1-1 *The Cycle of Violence*[19]*

- *Phase or Stage One:* Tension mounts, and the victim makes increased efforts to please the abuser in hopes of avoiding violence. The victim who has been through the cycle repeatedly may actually attempt to antagonize the abuser, because he or she may feel that violence is inevitable and the tension causes increased stress.
- *Phase or Stage Two:* Violence erupts. Violence may be physical, verbal, or emotional, but it is always painful.
- *Phase or Stage Three:* The abuser apologizes for the violence and may show remorse, shame, or guilt. At this time the abuser is likely to promise to change or make concessions for the explosion with gifts and positive behavior. This is the stage of the relationship in which the victim may feel rewarded. Both partners may believe that the violence was self-limiting.

Modified from Walker LE: *The battered woman,* New York, 1979, Harper & Row.
*The cycle becomes shorter and shorter the more often it is repeated.

Box 1-2	*Examples of Why People Stay in Abusive Relationships*

- Fear for personal safety, safety of children, or safety of other family members
- Concern regarding economic issues (homelessness; childcare; employment; assets [investments, checking, and saving accounts], medical insurance, and car in partner's name)
- Feelings for the batterer—she still loves him or believes he can change
- Cultural and religious norms
- For immigrant women, fear of deportation or uncertainty of legal rights
- Family pressure to stay in the relationship
- Uncertainty of viable options, especially for women with children

CLINICAL CLUES

Many health care professionals fail to recognize signs of acute or recurrent violence. Health care providers need to be able to recognize the signs of IPV. These signs may vary depending on the type of abuse (i.e., emotional, financial, physical, or sexual), but some general guidelines should be used as a routine part of the assessment.

The first step for primary care providers would be medical record review from previous visits. Care providers should examine the medical record for signs and symptoms of injuries and medical complaints that form a pattern indicating domestic violence. While emergency room physicians rarely have an opportunity to do a medical record review, they may identify some of the indicators of abuse while discussing the patient's past medical history. Clinical indicators from the record review and patient history are included in Box 1-3

Because emergency room physicians operate in an acute or crisis orientation they frequently rely on direct observation of the patient for signs and symptoms of domestic violence. The American College of Emergency Physicians,[72] in its position statement in January 1998, reminds clinicians that the clinical findings listed in Box 1-4 should prompt direct questioning about domestic violence.

Box 1-3	*Clinical Indicators of Abuse From Medical Record Review or Patient History*

- Previous medical visits for injuries that were unexplained or for which illogical explanations were provided
- Multiple visits for anxiety-related concerns, including complaints of insomnia
- Patient concerns for pain related to headaches or pelvic, back, or chest pain
- Patient complaints of a choking sensation
- Past history of suicide attempts, depression, and substance use
- Erratic patient attendance—canceled appointments, showing up without an appointment, repeated emergency department visits
- Past record of breast and genital trauma or mutilation; burns; musculoskeletal damage (including broken bones); bruising on upper arms, face, and neck, and mouth and dental trauma; clumps of missing hair[77]
- Past history of soft tissue injuries, facial injuries, fractured teeth, perforated eardrums[39]
- Patient observations of excessive compliance, defiance, evasive answers, or passive/submissive behavior[68]
- Past pregnancy history of unwanted pregnancies and abortions; preterm deliveries; repeated sexually transmitted infections; positive toxicology screens; low-birth-weight infants; first or second trimester bleeding; delayed or inadequate care; repeated triage visits in labor and delivery; and missed appointments[36, 77]

Box 1-4	*Potential Indicators for Domestic Violence*

- Central pattern of injuries
- Contusions or injuries in the head, neck, or chest
- Injuries that suggest a defensive posture
- Types or extent of injuries that are inconsistent with the patient's explanation
- Substantial delay between when the injury occurred and when the patient came for treatment
- Injuries during pregnancy
- Pattern of repeated visits to the emergency department
- Evidence of alcohol or drug use
- Arriving in the emergency department as a result of a suicide attempt or rape
- Evasiveness, embarrassment, and lack of concern with the injuries
- A partner who is overly solicitous, answers questions for the patient, is hostile, defensive or aggressive, or who sets up communication barriers

From American College of Emergency Physicians: *Domestic violence,* Dallas, 1998, The College.

VIOLENCE SCREENING PROTOCOLS

Although review of the medical record and patient history provides indicators of abuse, other victims, not fitting the profile may not be screened; opportunities for both assessment and intervention are lost if health care providers rely only on indicators to identify patients for screening.[49] The American College of Obstetrics and Gynecology (ACOG) was the first national medical organization to advocate routine screening of all patients for intimate partner violence. ACOG and The Family Violence Prevention Fund, as well as other major national health organizations, have identified that screening should occur during initial and annual examinations, all patient care visits related to injury or trauma, and at least once a trimester in prenatal care.[39-41] Other national health care organizations, including the American Academy of Nurse Practitioners, the American Nurses Association, and the American Dental Association, have position statements regarding intimate partner violence. Members can refer to the individual website or call for a hard copy of the position statement desired. For a list of some of these organizations, including websites and phone numbers, refer to Appendix A.

The Family Violence Prevention Fund[41] also recommends that routine screening for domestic violence be done in the emergency department for all females older than 14 years. This screening should be done during every emergency department visit and should focus on abuse occurring over the past year. Screening should be carried out in private settings using straightforward, nonjudgmental questions and in a culturally competent manner. Documentation of screening outcomes should be confidential. Screening should be conducted by health care providers who have adequate education regarding domestic violence including cultural competency.* They should be trained in both how to ask questions and how to intervene. The screener must be someone authorized to record in the main body of the patient's medical record. Ideally, the screener should have a relationship of trust with the patient or, if not, a clearly defined role relating to domestic violence. Screening should be part of a face-to-face encounter. Professional interpreters rather than family members or friends should be used when there is a language barrier. When possible, the screening should be part of a written health questionnaire in the patient's native language.

Although individuals rarely consider themselves "abused," they will often admit to a specific type of assault. General guidelines for screening include using specific terms for abuse ("Have you been hit, slapped, kicked . . ." as opposed to "Are you a victim of or experiencing domestic violence"). Other significant components of screening are privacy and confidentiality. No one should be screened for domestic violence if he or she is accompanied by anyone, including children over the age of 3 or family members who serve as translators, parents, or friends. Patients must be told what the care provider will do with the information from the screen. State laws and institutional and personal practices for reporting domestic abuse should be reviewed so that women can develop trust in their health care providers.[68] See Box 1-5 for recommended screening questions, as well as a nonthreatening introduction to the topic.[20]

---

*Refer to Chapter 11 for more information about domestic violence and culture.

Box 1-5	*Screening Questions*

Domestic violence screening can be conducted by making the following statement and asking these three simple questions.

Because violence is so common in many women's lives and because there is help available for women being abused, I now ask every patient about domestic violence:

- Within the past year—or since you have been pregnant—have you been hit, slapped, kicked, or otherwise physically hurt by someone?
- Are you in a relationship with a person who threatens or physically hurts you?
- Has anyone forced you to have sexual activities that made you feel uncomfortable?

The Family Violence Prevention Fund's website (http://www.endabuse.org) also contains excellent examples of screening questions, as well as a multitude of related tools for clinicians across health care settings. See Appendix B for more screening and assessment tools.

From Family Violence Prevention Fund: *Preventing domestic violence: clinical guidelines on routine screening,* San Francisco, 1999, The Fund.

Intervention

One of the barriers that physicians have frequently identified to screening for domestic violence is lack of knowledge of how to intervene when patients acknowledge abuse. Several approaches to screening and intervening have been developed for health care providers to tackle this important task. For example, the Philadelphia Family Violence Working Group developed a domestic violence training program for physicians featuring a general approach that they presented with the acronym *RADAR* (*R*outinely screen female patients, *A*sk direct questions, *D*ocument your findings, *A*ssess patient safety, *R*eview options and make referrals).[73]

The intervention process follows an affirmative response to the violence screen. Health care providers can conduct the intervention themselves or refer to an in-house Licensed Social Worker or an Advocate from the local Battered Women's Shelter. Leigh Kimberg, MD found that she was able to provide the necessary interventions for her abused patients by dialing the number for the local Abuse Hotline connected with the shelter system and telling the patient that she wanted her to get the best possible information by talking with someone who can help her to keep safe. She suggests that this a time-sensitive way to provide appropriate care for abused patients.[74] If the health care provider is conducting the intervention, the first priority should be assessing patient safety; Campbell's Danger Assessment[75,76] reviewed in Box 1-6 is the most commonly used approach to help abused patients come to terms with the various aspects of violence within their life. After discussing the patient's current level of safety she should be asked if it is safe for her to go home when she leaves. If she responds negatively, immediate referral should be made to the local battered women's shelter. The next step in the intervention process is to offer other options that the patient can take to increase her safety level if she is not planning to go to a shelter. Alternatives include the development of a safety plan, obtaining a protection order, joining a support group organized by the local shelter, or talking to an advocate. Discussing possible ways to keep safe is

Box 1-6	*Danger Assessment*

Several risk factors have been associated with homicides (murders) of both batterers and battered women in research conducted after the murders have taken place. We cannot predict what will happen in your case, but we would like you to be aware of the danger of homicide in situations of severe battering and for you to see how many of the risk factors apply to your situation.

Using the calendar, please mark the approximate dates during the past year when you were beaten by your husband or partner. Write on that date how bad the incident was according to the following scale:

1. Slapping, pushing; no injuries and/or lasting pain
2. Punching, kicking; bruises, cuts, and/or continuing pain
3. "Beating up"; severe contusions, burns, broken bones
4. Threat to use weapon; head injury, internal injury, permanent injury
5. Use of weapon; wounds from weapon

(If **any** of the descriptions for the higher number apply, use the higher number.)

Mark **Yes** or **No** for each of the following. ("He" refers to your husband, partner, ex-husband, ex-partner, or whoever is currently physically hurting you.)

____ 1. Has the physical violence increased in severity or frequency over the past year?
____ 2. Has he ever used a weapon against you or threatened you with a weapon?
____ 3. Does he ever try to choke you?
____ 4. Does he own a gun?
____ 5. Has he ever forced you to have sex when you did not wish to do so?
____ 6. Does he use drugs? By drugs, I mean "uppers" or amphetamines, speed, angel dust, cocaine, "crack," street drugs or mixtures.
____ 7. Does he threaten to kill you and/or do you believe he is capable of killing you?
____ 8. Is he drunk every day or almost every day? (In terms of quantity of alcohol.)
____ 9. Does he control most or all of your daily activities? For instance: does he tell you who you can be friends with, when you can see your family, how much money you can use, or when you can take the car? (If he tries, but you do not let him, check here: ____)
____10. Have you ever been beaten by him while you were pregnant? (If you have never been pregnant by him, check here: ____)
____11. Is he violently and constantly jealous of you? (For instance, does he say "If I can't have you, no one can.")
____12. Have you ever threatened or tried to commit suicide?
____13. Has he ever threatened or tried to commit suicide?
____14. Does he threaten to harm your children?
____15. Do you have a child that is not his?
____16. Is he unemployed?
____17. Have you left him during the past year? (If you have *never* lived with him, check here____.)
____18. Do you currently have another (different) intimate partner?
____19. Does he follow or spy on you, leave threatening notes, destroy your property, or call you when you don't want him to?

____Total "Yes" Answers

Thank you. Please talk to your physician, nurse, advocate, or counselor about what the Danger Assessment means in terms of your situation.

Jacquelyn C. Campbell, Ph.D., R.N. Copyright 1985, 1988, 2001
Used with permission of the author.[75,76]

Box 1-7 *Safety Plan*	

• Hide money
• Hide an extra set of house and car keys
• Establish a code with family and friends
• Ask a neighbor to call the police if violence begins
• Hide a bag with extra clothing
	• Have available
	  • Social Security numbers (his, yours, children's)
	  • Birth certificates (yours and children's)
	  • Marriage license
	  • Driver's license
	  • Bank account numbers
	  • Insurance policies and numbers
	  • Rent and utility receipts
	  • Important phone numbers

From McFarlane J, Gondolf E: Preventing abuse during pregnancy: a clinical protocol, *Am J Matern Child Nurs* 23:26, 1998.

an essential aspect of the intervention including referrals to appropriate community agencies (Legal Aid, Victim's Assistance, Battered Women's Shelters) and the development of a Safety Plan[77] (Box 1-7).

Documentation

When domestic violence is discovered during the patient interview or examination, appropriate documentation is required to ensure that the medical record is useful during any legal proceedings, either criminal or civil. Various published tools are available that can assist the clinician document history of abuse, extent of injury, and associated symptoms. Although there is no single format for documenting abuse, all patient records should include the following:
- Photographs of injuries, as well as body maps (each should correspond to the other).
- Specific written injury description, including size, shape, location, quality of injury, foreign bodies.
- Clearly identifiable patient quotes, including specifics of the incident (i.e., offender relationship, location and time of assault, mechanisms of injury). Patient statements should not be summarized.

A summary of important information for screening and intervening in domestic violence is presented in Box 1-8.

Professional role involvement in policy making arenas as well as local coalitions increase health care providers' abilities to influence legislation on program and research funding, gun laws, and child abuse concerns.[78] Clinical involvement with victims of abuse can be intense, stressful work. Health care providers need to care for themselves by clearly identifying their goals in screening and intervening and by casting themselves in a role of providing referral and assistance as opposed to assuming the "rescuer" position.[74] Working with local violence coalitions can enhance knowledge of local resources and provide a common ground to share concerns and frustrations with other professionals who have similar struggles.

Box 1-8	*Health Care Providers Implications for Caring for Women Experiencing Violence*

ASSESS

- *Set the stage:* Use environmental prompts that indicate your interest in domestic violence to your clinical population. Wear pins that say "You can talk to me about family violence" and put posters in clinical areas and in women's bathrooms about domestic violence and local resources. Leave safety cards with resource information and phone numbers in examination rooms and in bathrooms for women to take home with them.
- *Ask privately:* Do not ask when anyone else is in the room, including parents, partners, children over the age of 3, "girlfriends," or family members.
- *Be honest:* Describe why you are asking about domestic violence and what you will be doing with the information. Become familiar with state laws about reporting domestic violence. Women need to know what you will and will not report.
- *Be complete:* Ask about physical abuse ("Have you been hit, slapped, kicked, or otherwise physically hurt by anyone?" "Who?"). Remember to ask about additional perpetrators with teens ("Who else?"). Ask about emotional abuse ("Are you afraid of anyone?"). Ask about forced sex ("Has anyone forced you into having sex or becoming intimate against your will?"). Remember that the perpetrator might be a female.
- Ask how the person copes or keeps safe from violence. Listen for instances of use of substances, unsafe exercise, and isolating strategies. Are their children in the household at risk for harm?

INTERVENE

- Provide information about community agencies.
- Assure the woman that you will not reveal information about her violence experiences with her family or perpetrator. Keep the chart and abuse documentation in a secure area isolated from visitors. Tell her that you will treat her perpetrator like any other family member so that you will not jeopardize her safety.
- Help her to identify trusted individuals that she can approach for assistance.
- Develop a safety plan by working with the woman and incorporating her ideas.
- Tell her that she can contact the hospital, clinic, or doctor's office for assistance between visits.

DOCUMENT

- Include information in the chart with as many direct quotes as possible from the teen. Describe specific information about suggested resources and safety planning discussed during the interaction. Use a body map and photographs if there are bruises or scars present. Record the safety plan and referrals given to the woman.

EVALUATE

- Tell the woman that you and other health care providers will ask her in subsequent visits about her safety. Refer to information in her medical record to inquire about her success in developing a safety plan and contacting community resources.
- Celebrate each step taken as a step toward keeping safe.

Modified from Renker PR: Keeping safe: teenagers' strategies for dealing with perinatal violence, *JOGNN* 32(1):663-672, 2003

SUMMARY AND CONCLUSION

Today, domestic violence is widely seen as a significant public health issue. The number of clinicians who are regularly and appropriately screening for domestic violence has increased and many medical and nursing education programs include information about domestic violence in their curricula. However, after screening, many clinicians are at a loss for what should be done when domestic violence is identified. Beyond handing out shelter phone numbers, many are unsure of how to approach the situation, particularly if the patient has no intention of immediately leaving the assailant. Frequently, a patient's refusal to leave the violent situation halts further assistance from the health care arena. In some instances, it may trigger punitive action, such as threatening to have children removed from the home.

Understanding why people stay in violent relationships and how to keep them safe in the context of their individual situations is key for all clinicians. Identifying key community and interagency resources up front ensures that no one need care for victims of violence in a vacuum. A strong team approach, including multiple disciplines, will result in the most appropriate, personalized care for patients experiencing violence in their lives. It will also promote coalition building among community members, as individuals begin to recognize the role each plays in working with victims of domestic violence.

REFERENCES

1. Rennison CM, Welchans S: *Intimate partner violence,* Washington, DC, 2000, Bureau of Justice Statistics.
2. Tjadenn P, Thoennes N: *Full report of the prevalence, incidence and consequences of intimate partner violence,* Washington, DC, 2000, National Institute of Justice and Centers for Disease Control and Prevention.
3. Arias I, Pape K: Psychological abuse: implications for adjustment and commitment to leave violent partners, *Violence Vict* 14(1):55-67, 1999.
4. Canterino J and others: Domestic abuse in pregnancy: a comparison of self-completed domestic abuse questionnaire with a directed interview, *Am J Obstet Gynecol* 181:1049-1051, 1999.
5. Cokkinides V, Coker A, Sanderson M: Physical violence during pregnancy: maternal complications and birth outcomes, *Obstet Gynecol* 93:661-666, 1999.
6. Martin SL: Physical abuse of women before, during, and after pregnancy, *JAMA* 285:1581-1584, 2001.
7. McGrath ME, Hogan JW, Peipert JF: A prevalence survey of abuse and screening for abuse in urgent care of patients, *Obstet Gynecol* 91:511-514, 1998.
8. Shumway J and others: Preterm labor, placental abruption, and premature rupture of membranes in relation to maternal violence or verbal abuse, *J Matern Fetal Med* 8(3):76-80, 1999.
9. Torres S and others: Abuse during and before pregnancy: prevalence and cultural correlates, *Violence Vict* 15:303-321, 2000.
10. Centers for Disease Control and Prevention: Building data systems for monitoring and responding to violence against women: recommendations from a workshop, *MMWR* 49(RR11):2000.
11. Saltzman LE and others: *Intimate partner violence surveillance uniform definitions and recommended data elements,* Atlanta, 1999, Center for Disease Control and Prevention National Center of Injury Prevention and Control.
12. Plichta SB, Falik M: 2001 Prevalence of violence and it's implications for women's health, *Women's Health Issues* 11:244-258, 2001.
13. Straus M: Measuring interfamily conflict and violence: The Conflict Tactics (CT) Scale, *J Marriage Family* 41:75-86, 1979.
14. Tollestrup K and others: Health indicators and intimate partner violence among women who are members of a managed care organization, *Prevent Med* 29:431-440, 1999.

15. Tolman RM: The development of a measure of psychological maltreatment of women by their male partners, *Violence Vict* 51:159-177, 1989,

16. Hedin LW, Janson PO: The invisible wounds: the occurrence of psychological abuse and anxiety compared with previous experience of physical abuse during the childbearing years, *J Psychosomatic Obstet Gynecol* 20(3):136-144, 1999.

17. Hudson W, McIntosh S: The index of spouse abuse: two identifiable dimensions, *J Marriage Family* 43:873-888, 1981.

18. Dutton DG, Golant SK: *The batterer: a psychological profile,* New York, 1995, Basic Books.

19. Walker LE: *The battered woman,* New York, 1979, Harper & Row.

20. Frank J, Rodowski M: Review of psychological issues in victims of domestic violence seen in emergency room settings, *Emerg Med Clin North Am* 17(3):657-677, 1999.

21. Marshall L: Development of the severity of violence against women scales, *J Fam Viol* 7:103-121, 1992.

22. Parker B and others: Physical and emotional abuse in pregnancy: a comparison of adult and teenage women, *Nurs Res* 42:173-178, 1993.

23. Follingstad D and others: The role of emotional abuse in physically abusive relationships, *J Family Violence* 5:107-120, 1990.

24. Sackett LA, Saunders DG: The impact of different forms of psychological abuse on battered women, *Violence Vict* 14(1):105-117, 1999.

25. Haggerty LA and others: Pregnant women's perceptions of abuse, *JOGNN* 3(3):283-290, 2001.

26. Smith PH, Earp J, DeVellis R: Measuring battering: development of the Women's Experience with Battering (WEB) Scale, *Women's Health* 1:273-288: 1995.

27. Smith PH, Tessaro I, Earp JL: Women's experiences with battering: a conceptualization from qualitative research, *Women's Health Issues* 5:173-182, 1995.

28. Wiemann CM and others: Pregnant adolescents: experiences and behaviors associated with physical assault by an intimate partner, *Matern Child Health J* 4(2):93-101, 2000.

29. Campbell JC, Alford P: The dark consequences of marital rape, *Am J Nurs* 89:946-949, 1989.

30. Evins G, Chescheir N: Prevalence of domestic violence among women seeking abortion services, *Women's Health Issues* 6:204-210, 1996.

31. Parker B, McFarlane J, Soeken K: Abuse during pregnancy: effects on maternal complications and birth weight in adults and teenage women, *Obstet Gynecol* 170:323-328, 1994.

32. Jacoby M and others: Rapid repeat pregnancy and experiences of interpersonal violence among low-income adolescents, *Am J Prevent Med* 16:318-320, 1999.

33. Campbell J and others: Correlates of battering during pregnancy, *Res Nurs Health* 15:229-236, 1992.

34. Gazmarian J and others: Violence and reproductive health: current knowledge and future research directions, *Matern Child Health J* 4(2):79-83, 2000.

35. McFarlane J, Parker B, Soeken K: Abuse during pregnancy: associations with maternal health and infant birthweight, *Nurs Res* 45:37-42, 1996.

36. Renker P: Physical abuse, social support, self care, and pregnancy outcomes of older adolescents, *JOGNN* 28:377-388, 1999.

37. Curry M, Doyle B, Gilhooley J: Abuse among pregnant adolescents: differences by developmental age, *Am J Matern Child Nurs* 23(3):144-150, 1999.

38. Durant T and others: Opportunities for intervention: discussing physical abuse during prenatal care visits, *Am J Prevent Med* 19(4):238-244, 2000.

39. American College of Obstetricians and Gynecologists: *Domestic violence,* Technical Bulletin 209:1-9, 1995.

40. American Medical Association, Council on Ethical and Judicial Affairs: Physicians and domestic violence: ethical considerations, *JAMA* 267:3190-3193, 1992.

41. Family Violence Prevention Fund: *Preventing domestic violence: clinical guidelines on routine screening,* San Francisco, 1999, The Fund.

42. Chamberlain L: Your words make a difference: broader implications for screening, *Family Violence Prevention Fund Health Alert* 7(1):1-4.

43. Chamberlain L, Perham-Hester K: Physician screening practices for female partner abuse during prenatal visits, *Matern Child Health J* 4:141-147, 2000.

44. Horan DL and others: Domestic violence screening practices of obstetrician-gynecology patients for domestic violence, *Am J Obstet Gynecol* 92(5):785-789, 1998.
45. Renker P: Keep a blank face: I need to tell you what has been happening to me: teens' strategies for dealing with perinatal violence, *Am J Matern Child Nurs* 27(2):109-116, 2002
46. Waalen J and others: Screening for intimate partner violence by health care providers: barriers and interventions, *Am J Prevent Med* 19:230-237, 2000.
47. Caralis P, Musialowski R: Women's experiences with domestic violence and their attitudes and expectations regarding medical care of abuse victims, *South Med J* 90:1075-1080, 1997.
48. Parsons LH and others: Methods and attitudes toward screening obstetrics and gynecology patients for domestic violence, *Am J Obstet Gynecol* 173:381-386, 1995.
49. Rodriguez MA and others: Screening and intervention for intimate partner abuse practices and attitudes of primary care physicians, *JAMA* 282:468-474,1999.
50. Smith PH, Davis M, Helmick L: Changing the health care response to battered women: a health education approach, *Family Community Health* 20(4):1-18,1998.
51. Clark K and others: Who gets screened during pregnancy for partner violence? *Arch Family Med* 9:1093-1099, 2000.
52. Collins KS and others: *Health concerns across a woman's life span: the Commonwealth Fund 1998 survey of women's health,* New York, 1999, The Commonwealth Fund.
53. National Institute of Justice and Centers for Disease Control and Prevention: *Prevalence, incidence and consequences of violence against women: findings from the National Violence Against Women Survey,* Washington, DC, 1998, The Institute and The Centers.
54. Campbell JC and others: Battered women's experience in the emergency department, *J Emerg Nurs* 20(4):280-288, 1994.
55. McFarlane J and others: Identification of abuse in emergency departments: effectiveness of a two-question tool, *J Emerg Nurs* 21(5):391-394, 1995.
56. Feldhaus KM and others: Accuracy of three brief screening questions for detecting partner violence in the emergency department, *JAMA* 277(17):1357-1361, 1997.
57. Dearwater SR et al: Prevalence of intimate partner abuse in women treated at community hospital emergency departments, *JAMA* 280(5):433-438, 1998.
58. Goldberg WG: Tomlanovich MD, Domestic violence victims in the emergency department, *JAMA* 251(24):3259-3264, 1984.
59. Covington D and others: Poor hospital documentation of violence against women, *J Trauma* 38(3):412-416, 1995.
60. Gremillion DH, Kanof EP: Overcoming barriers to physician involvement in identifying and referring victims of domestic violence, *Ann Emerg Med* 27(6):769-773, 1996.
61. Gerbert B and others: When asked, patients tell: disclosure of sensitive health risk behaviors, *Med Care* 37(1):104-111, 1999.
62. Rodriguez MA, Quiroga SS, Bauer HM: Breaking the silence: battered women's perspectives on medical care, *Arch Family Med* 5:153-158, 1996.
63. Glass N, Campbell JC: Mandatory reporting of intimate partner violence by health care professionals: a policy review, *Nurs Outlook* 46(6):279-283, 1998.
64. Hayden SR, Barton ED, Hayden M: Domestic violence in the emergency department: how do women prefer to disclose and discuss issues? *J Emerg Med* 15:447-451.
65. McCauley J, Kern D, Kolodner K: Clinical characteristics of women with a history of childhood abuse, *JAMA* 277:1362-1368, 1998.
66. Rodriquez MA and others: Patient attitudes about mandatory reporting of domestic violence: implications for general health care professionals, *West J Med* 169:337-341, 1998.
67. Yam M, Oradell NJ: Seen but not heard: battered women's perceptions of the ED experience, *J Emerg Nurs* 26:464-470, 2000.
68. Renker P: *Keeping safe: health care professionals' contributions and missed steps in helping teens to keep safe from perinatal violence.* Paper presented at Lighting the Way, The 2002 Conference of The American Association of Women's Health, Obstetrical, and Neonatal Nurses. June 25, 2002.

69. Gerbert B and others: How health care providers help battered women: the survivor's perspective, *Women Health* 29(3):115-135, 1999.
70. Campbell J: Abuse during pregnancy: progress, policy and potential. *Am J Public Health* 88:185-187, 1998.
71. Coker A and others: Frequency and correlates of intimate partner violence by type: physical, sexual, and psychological battering, *Am J Public Health* 90:553-559, 2000.
72. American College of Emergency Physicians: *Domestic violence,* 1998, The College.
73. Harwell TS and others: Results of a domestic violence training program offered to the staff of urban community health centers: Evaluation Committee of the Philadelphia Family Violence Working Group, *Am J Prevent Med* 15:235-242, 1998.
74. Kimberg L: Screening for domestic violence changed my practice. Family Violence Prevention Fund Health Alert, *Family Violence Prevention Fund* 6(2):1-3,1999.
75. Campbell J: Assessment of risk of homicide for battered women, *Adv Nurs Sci* 8(4):36-51, 1986.
76. Campbell J: *Assessing dangerousness: violence by sexual offenders, batterers, and child abusers,* Thousand Oaks, Calif, 1995, Sage.
77. McFarlane J, Gondolf E: Preventing abuse during pregnancy: a clinical protocol, *Am J Matern Child Nurs* 23:22-27, 1998.
78. Fontanarosa PB: The unrelenting epidemic of violence in America: truths and consequences, *JAMA* 273(22):1792-1793, 1995.
79. Merrill J: Social support for victims of domestic violence, *J Psychosoc Nurs* 39(11):30-35, 2001.

2 INJURY PATTERNS AND PATTERNED INJURIES

Jenifer Markowitz • S. Scott Polsky • David Effron

It is important to look for patterns as clues to mechanisms of injury. Injuries can display either a distinct *injury pattern,* such as defensive wounds to the forearms, or *patterned injury,* such as ligature marks.[1] They can be quite distinctive and should be noted as explicitly as possible, preferably with photographs (Table 2-1, Figures 2-1 and 2-2).

One of the most common types of injuries, especially from blunt force trauma, is the contusion. The appearance and distribution of contusions can reveal quite a bit about the mechanism of injury, and any appearing on the body should be examined closely. However, attempts to characterize the age of contusions by color or other physical findings should not be undertaken.[2,3] The clinician must remember that contusions will not always be evident at the time of examination; this is especially true if the victim is seen soon after the assault. If there is suspicion that further injuries may become more apparent over time, consider having the patient return in 24 to 72 hours, so that further assessment and documentation can be completed (Figures 2-3 and 2-4).

Table 2-1	*Frequently Used Descriptors*
TERM	INJURY PATTERN
Abrasion	Wound produced by friction scraping away epidermis or disruption of epidermis by direct pressure or rubbing
Contusion	Bruise occurring as the result of hemorrhage into soft tissues resulting from rupture of blood vessels caused by blunt force injury
Hematoma	Focal collection of extravasated blood
Laceration	Tear of skin or tissue caused by stretching of tissue
Avulsion	Ripping of an appendage from the body as a result of direct force or a ripping of skin and soft tissue from underlying structures as a result of an oblique glancing blow
Stab wound	Sharp force injury in which the wound is deeper than it is long
Incised wound	Sharp force injury in which the wound is longer than it is deep
Chop wound	A sharp force injury that will also have blunt characteristics; usually resulting from heavy weapons with a cutting edge, such as axes or cleavers

Modified from Davis GJ: Pattern of injury: blunt and sharp, *Clin Lab Med* 18(1):339-350, 1998.

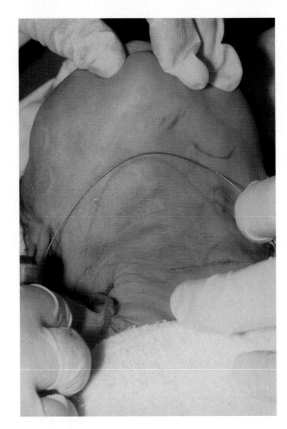

FIGURE 2-1 Multiple ligature marks from wire. *(Courtesy Dr. Elizabeth K. Balraj, Coroner Cuyahoga County, Cleveland, Ohio.)*

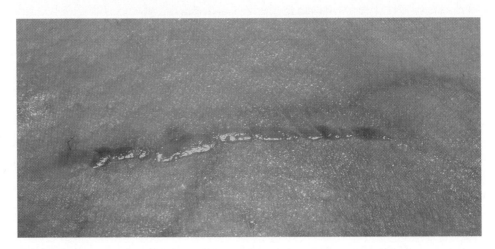

FIGURE 2-2 Ligature marks from wire. *(Courtesy Dr. Elizabeth K. Balraj, Coroner Cuyahoga County, Cleveland, Ohio.)*

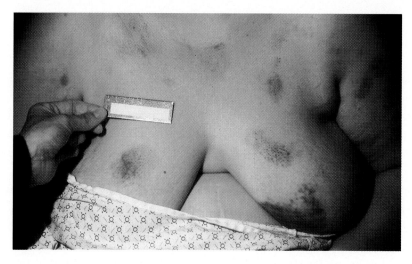

FIGURE 2-3   Multiple contusions following assault. *(Courtesy Dr. David Effron, MetroHealth Medical Center, Cleveland, Ohio.)*

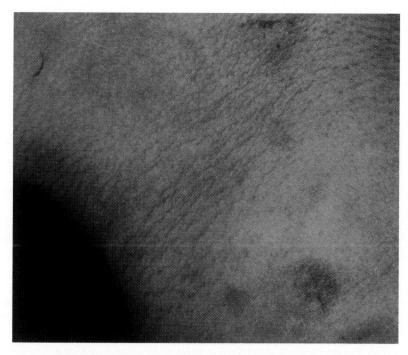

FIGURE 2-4   Fingertip contusions—note general uniformity of size of bruises. *(Courtesy Dr. Jenifer Markowitz, The DOVE Program, Summa Health System, Akron, Ohio.)*

Contusions will not always appear after blunt force. The absence of contusions does not negate the plausibility of the assault.[3] Bruising is very individual; amount of force, location of the injury, and amount of blood escaping into surrounding tissue can all affect the appearance of contusions. This is why it is difficult to accurately estimate the age of contusions based simply on appearance. It is also difficult to estimate the force of the trauma based solely on the appearance of contusions; lacerations, abrasions, and other injuries must be present to draw accurate conclusions.[2]

Other injuries such as lacerations (tearing injuries), slicing or cutting wounds (incisions), and deep, penetrating wounds (including chopping wounds) can also divulge a great deal of information about mechanism of injury (Figure 2-5). Special attention should be paid to any suspicious soft tissue injuries that could be secondary to a wielded object. Specific documentation of the size, shape, location, and coloration of the wound should be noted. Ideally, a photograph of the injury should be included in the patient's records, both before and after wound repair.

The hand is the most commonly used weapon in blunt force trauma secondary to domestic violence.[4] As with all essentially linear or flat objects, the hand often leaves distinctive soft tissue findings. The force of the blow is distributed to the tissue in a manner that displaces

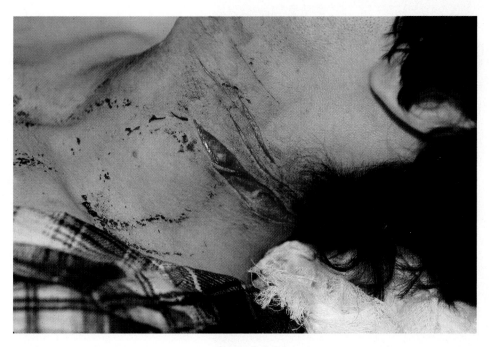

FIGURE 2-5   Neck   laceration.   *(Courtesy   Dr.   David   Effron,   MetroHealth   Medical   Center,*
Cleveland, Ohio.)

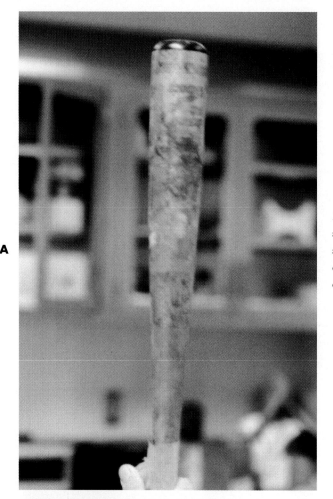

A

FIGURE 2-6 **A,** Injuries resulting from assault with a bat and the bat used. **B,** Note areas of central clearing caused by the impact of the bat. *(Courtesy Dr. Lisa Kohler, Summit County Medical Examiner, Akron, Ohio.)*

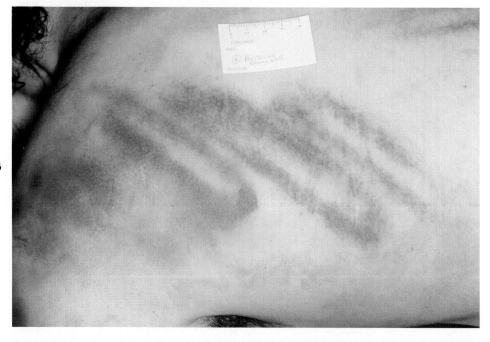

B

INJURY PATTERNS AND PATTERNED INJURIES

the impact and causes a central area of clearing surrounded by contusion. An open-handed blow therefore may be characterized by alternating linear contusions with central areas of clearing. With this mechanism in mind, other linear objects may be recognized (Figure 2-6). The object used as a weapon often leaves marks that correspond to the shape of the weapon. A club, asp, or board will show similar findings of contusion with central clearing adjusted to the size of the object. The impact of the corner of the weapon may also be recognized (Figures 2-7 through 2-13). Other distinctive markings caused by the hand as a weapon include the evenly spaced contusions with semicircular abrasions of fingernails (Figure 2-14) and the evenly spaced circular impacts from the knuckles of a closed fist.[4]

Text continued on page 32

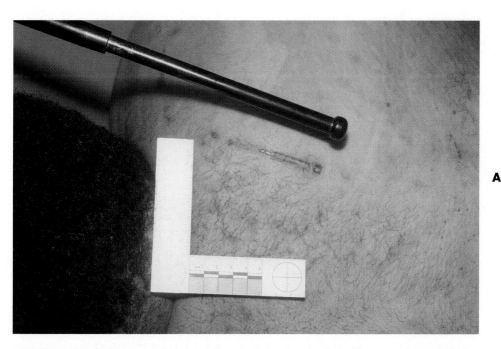

A

FIGURE 2-7 **A,** Linear contusions with central clearing resulting from assault with an asp. *(Courtesy Dr. Elizabeth K. Balraj, Coroner Cuyahoga County, Cleveland, Ohio.)* *Continued*

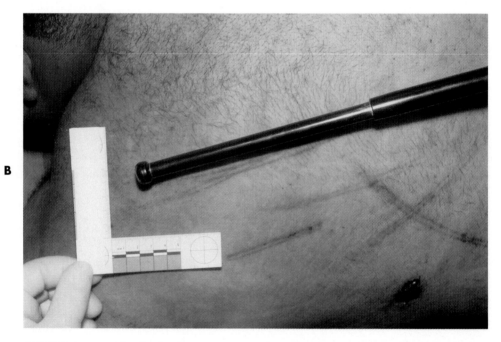

FIGURE 2-7, cont'd **B,** Matched contusion with asp handle. *(Courtesy Dr. Elizabeth K. Balraj, Coroner Cuyahoga County, Cleveland, Ohio.)*

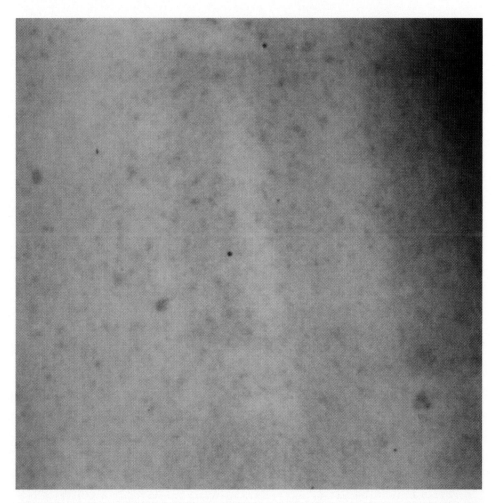

FIGURE 2-8   Patterned injury from assault with numchucks. *(Courtesy Dr. Jenifer Markowitz, The DOVE Program, Summa Health System, Akron, Ohio.)*

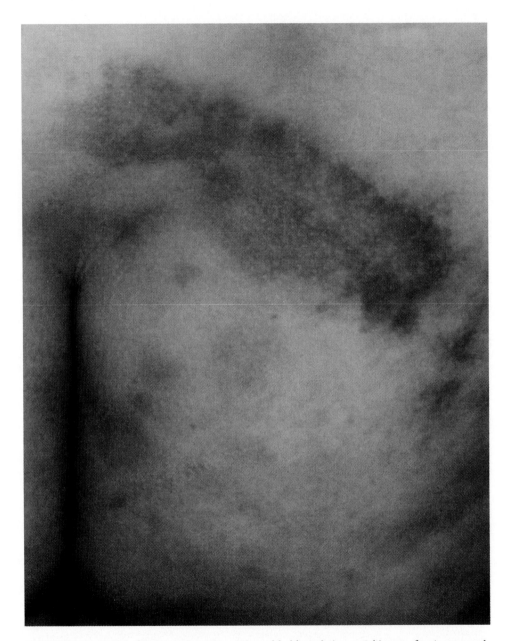

FIGURE 2-9   Injury from assault with a nail-studded board almost 24 hours after it occurred. Close attention reveals the nail clusters on the inferior aspect of the pattern, as well as the more obvious central clearing from the impact of the board. *(Courtesy Dr. Jenifer Markowitz, The DOVE Program, Summa Health System, Akron, Ohio.)*

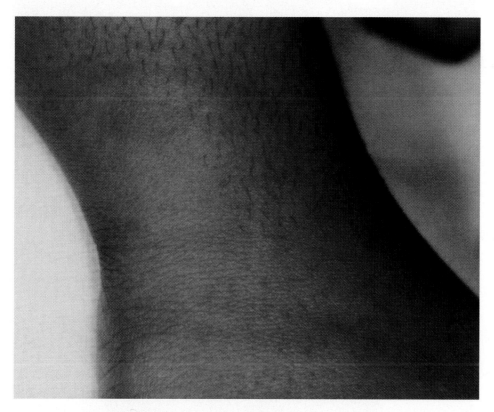

FIGURE 2-10   Whip marks resulting from assault with a cord. *(Courtesy Dr. Jenifer Markowitz, The DOVE Program, Summa Health System, Akron, Ohio.)*

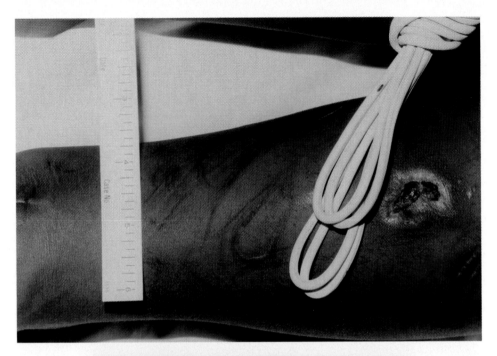

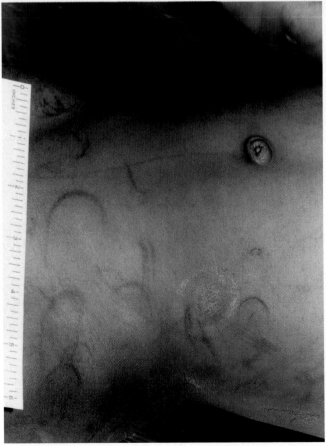

FIGURE 2-11 Curvilinear contusions resulting from assault with an electrical cord and the matching cord. *(Courtesy Dr. Elizabeth K. Balraj, Coroner Cuyahoga County, Cleveland, Ohio.)*

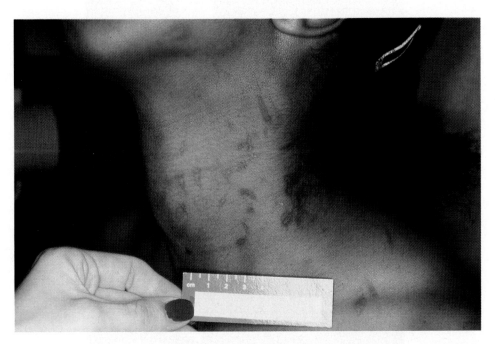

FIGURE 2-12   Marks made with a hairbrush. *(Courtesy Dr. David Effron, MetroHealth Medical Center, Cleveland, Ohio.)*

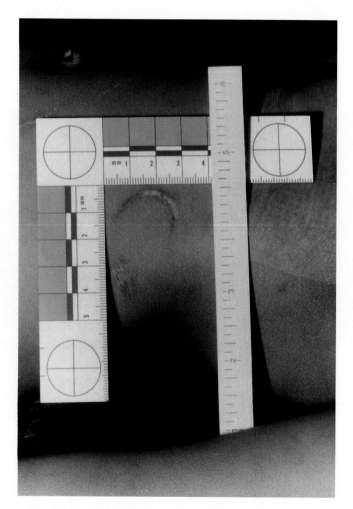

FIGURE 2-13 Imprint from a metal buckle. *(Courtesy Dr. Elizabeth K. Balraj, Coroner Cuyahoga County, Cleveland, Ohio.)*

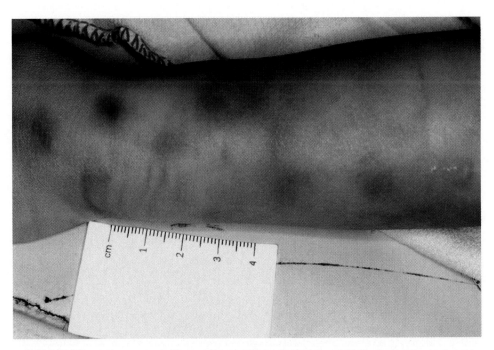

FIGURE 2-14   Multiple subtle fingertip contusions. *(Courtesy Dr. Lisa Kohler, Summit County Medical Examiner, Akron, Ohio.)*

The face, head, and neck are commonly the target of an attack. Studies examining locations of injury following interpersonal violence demonstrate that the majority of injuries incurred during an assault are craniofacial.[5,6] They may also provide clues about mechanisms of injury, especially in strangulation cases. Subconjunctival hemorrhaging may be evident after the strangling incident along with petechiae around the eyes, nose, mouth, and oral mucosa (Figures 2-15 and 2-16). Chin abrasions may also be evident, as a result of the victim struggling to break free of the assailant. Erythema may or may not be present and will not necessarily result in a contusion. Contusions that do appear will often display the pattern of the assailant's fingertips and may extend up to the chin and jaw line and down to the clavicles. If a ligature was used in the strangling event, marks may be evident reflecting the weapon used, such as telephone cords or rope. Presence of ligature marks should trigger further evaluation for a hyoid bone fracture.[7]

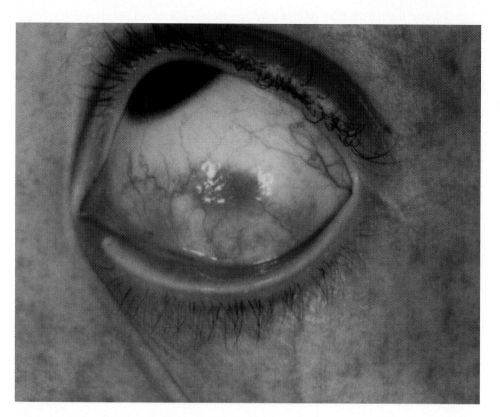

FIGURE 2-15 Petechial hemorrhage from attempted strangulation. *(Courtesy The DOVE Program, Summa Health System, Akron, Ohio.)*

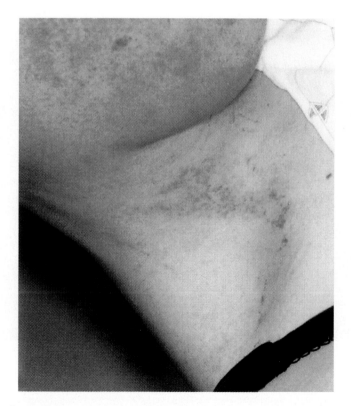

FIGURE 2-16   Petechial hemorrhage from strangulation. *(Courtesy The DOVE Program, Summa Health System, Akron, Ohio.)*

When the patient suffers direct blows to the face, patterned injuries may be noted as a result of the weapon used (Figure 2-17) as well as the victim's own accessories, such as a hat or eyeglasses. Figure 2-18 illustrates the specific pattern of injury corresponding to the edge of the patient's eyeglass frames. The foot is also a frequently used weapon. The shoe or boot often leaves characteristic marks that both help identify the cause of the injury and provide forensic evidence useful in prosecuting the assailant (Figures 2-19 through 2-21).

Text continued on page 39

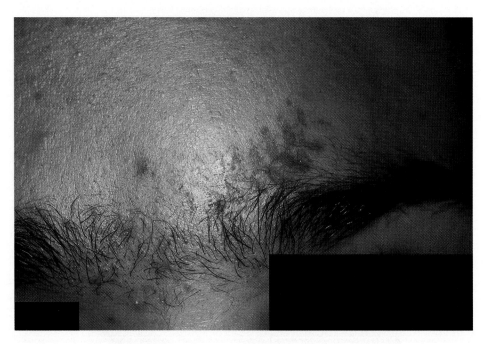

FIGURE 2-17   Face baseball stitching. *(Courtesy Dr. David Effron, MetroHealth Medical Center, Cleveland, Ohio.)*

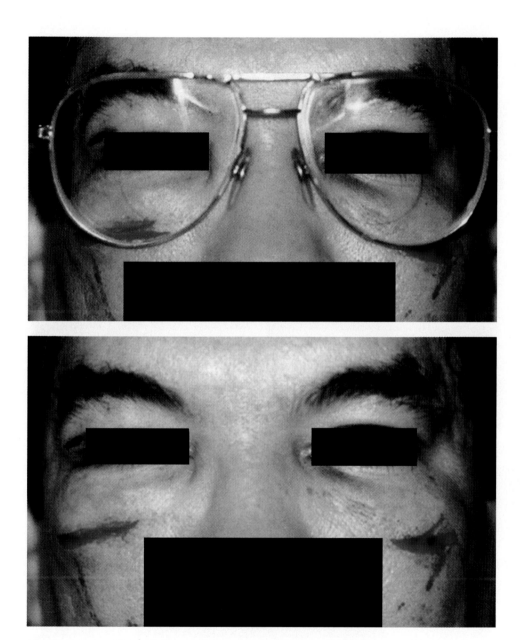

FIGURE 2-18   Glasses injury to the face. *(Courtesy Dr. David Effron, MetroHealth Medical Center, Cleveland, Ohio.)*

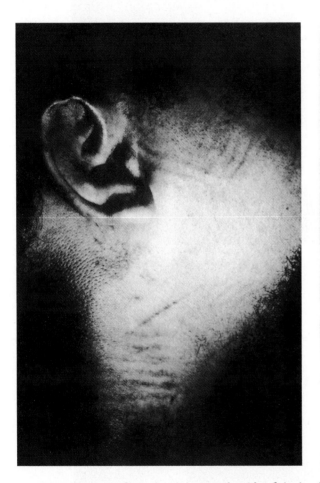 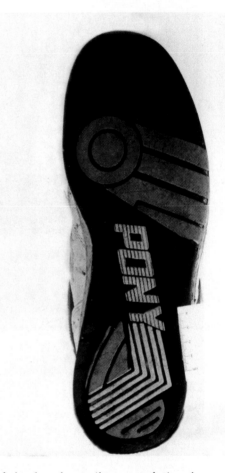

FIGURE 2-19 Stomping injury to the side of the head and the shoe the assailant wore during the assault. Note the distinctive pattern of the sole of the shoe and the matching pattern left on the victim's face. *(Courtesy Dr. Lisa Kohler, Summit County Medical Examiner, Akron, Ohio.)*

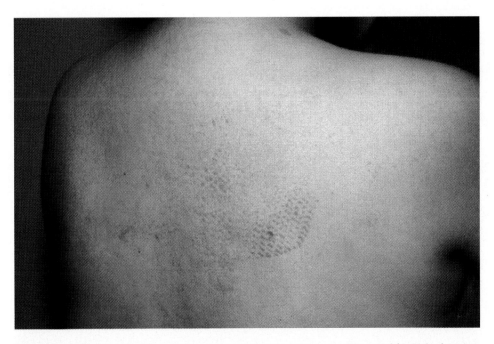

FIGURE 2-20 Sneaker imprint. *(Courtesy Dr. David Effron, MetroHealth Medical Center, Cleveland, Ohio.)*

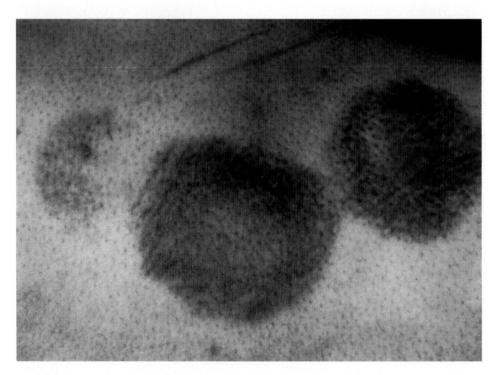

FIGURE 2-21 Bruising from a heavy workboot. This injury was a stomping injury, with the victim flat on the ground when it occurred. *(Courtesy Jill Bunnell, RNc, FNE, The DOVE Program, Summa Health System, Akron, Ohio.)*

Other soft tissue injuries consistent with abuse include bites, burns, or certain lacerations. A pair of matching semicircular, evenly spaced contusions may indicate a human bite.[1] Recognition of a bite wound not only may be important visually but also often yields saliva, which may be swabbed with a sterile cotton-tipped applicator moistened with sterile water or normal saline for evidentiary purposes[2] (Figures 2-22 through 2-25 on pp. 39-41). These contusions may have superficial abrasions, may be incomplete, or may show signs of pulling the appendage away during the incident.

Regardless of the type of weapon, all weapons have the capability of causing patterned injury. In some cases, the pattern will be more obvious than in others, as illustrated in Figures 2-26 through 2-28. Some patterned injuries will arise not as a result of the weapon itself but as a result of the weapon coming in contact with the patient's clothing, as seen in Figure 2-29.

Text continued on page 47

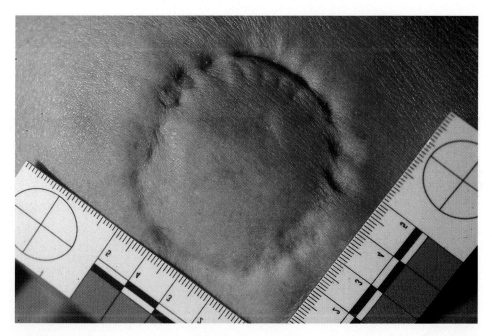

FIGURE 2-22   Bite impression. *(Courtesy Jill Bunnell, RNc, FNE, The DOVE Program, Summa Health System, Akron, Ohio.)*

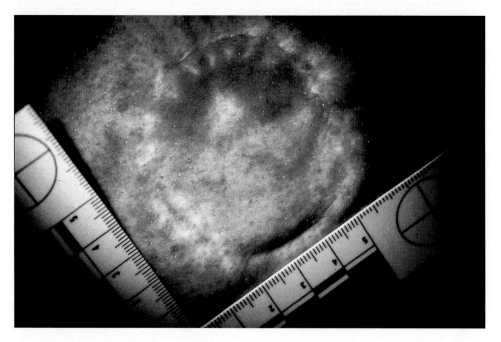

FIGURE 2-23 Bite impression from Figure 2-22, as seen with alternate light source. *(Courtesy Jill Bunnell, RNc, FNE, The DOVE Program, Summa Health System, Akron, Ohio.)*

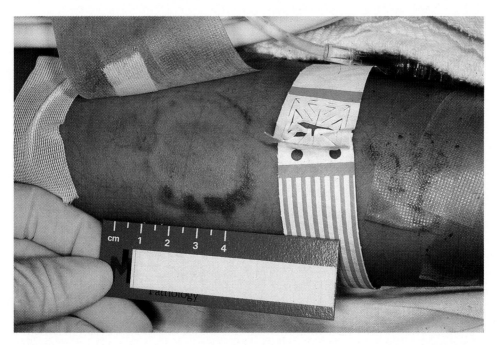

FIGURE 2-24   Bite mark on an adult. Arch form and width fairly distinguishable. *(Courtesy Dr. David Effron, MetroHealth Medical Center, Cleveland, Ohio.)*

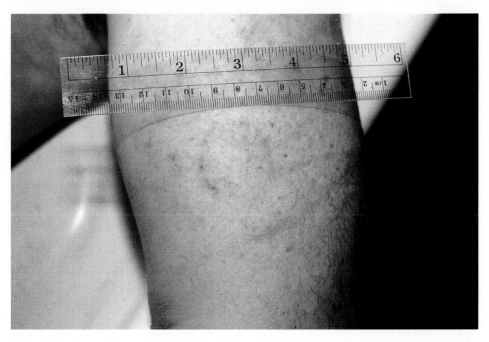

FIGURE 2-25   Healing bite wound. *(Courtesy Dr. E. Thomas Marshall Sr., DDS, Forensic Odontologist, Summit County Medical Examiner, Akron, Ohio.)*

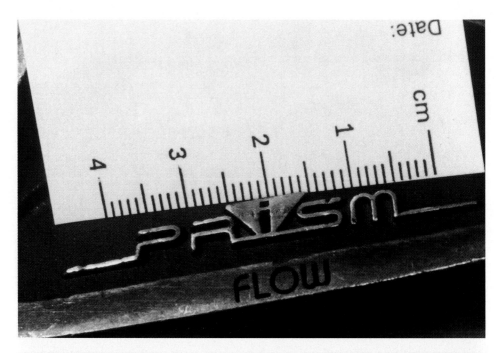

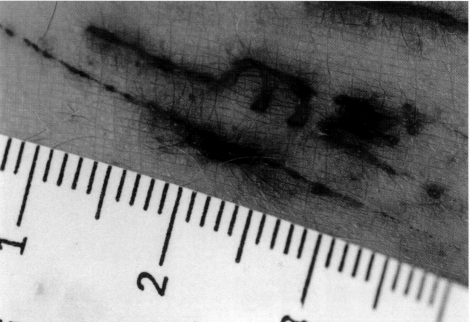

FIGURE 2-26   Detailing from a metal implement used in an assault and the resulting abrasion.
(Courtesy Dr. Lisa Kohler, Summit County Medical Examiner, Akron, Ohio.)

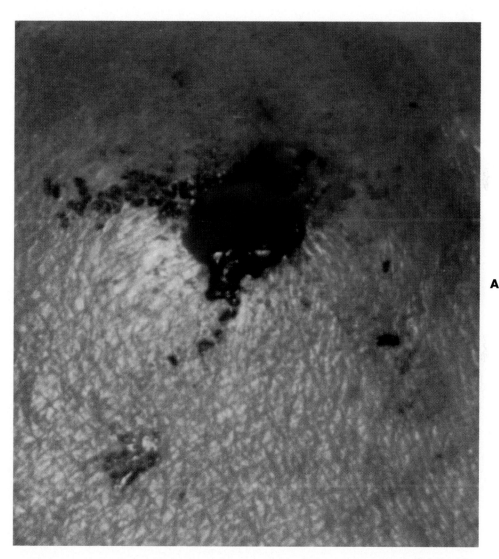

FIGURE 2-27   Injuries inflicted by a claw hammer. **A,** Blunt trauma to the skull resulting from the rounded end of the hammer. *(Courtesy Jill Bunnell, RNc, FNE, The DOVE Program, Summa Health System, Akron, Ohio.)*   *Continued*

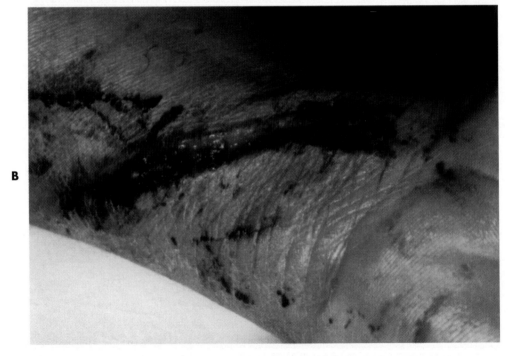

FIGURE 2-27, cont'd Injuries inflicted by a claw hammer. **B,** Defensive tearing injury from the claw end of the hammer.

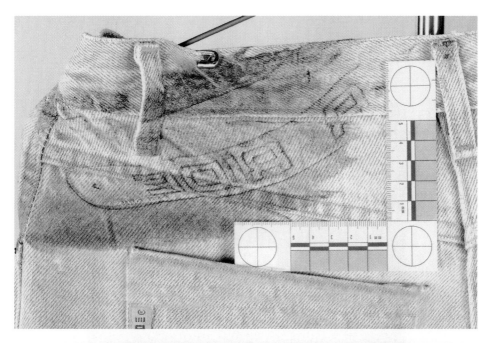

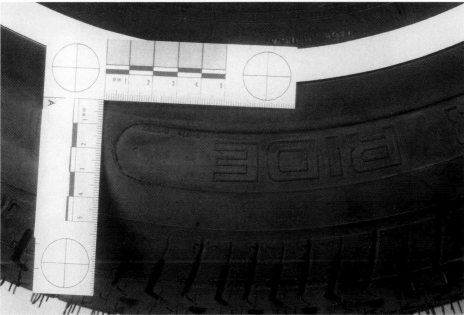

FIGURE 2-28 Tire marks on clothing. *(Courtesy Dr. Elizabeth K. Balraj, Coroner Cuyahoga County, Cleveland, Ohio.)*

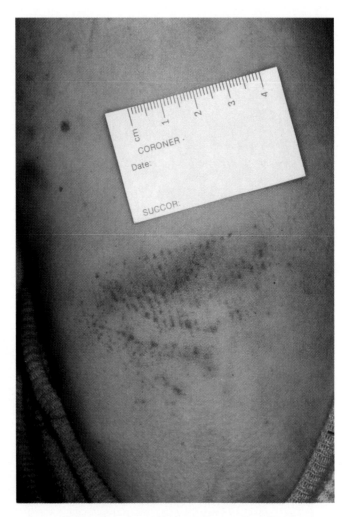

FIGURE 2-29   Patterned abrasion caused by victim's sweater. Although the sweater was not the weapon, its impact with the weapon caused the resulting patterned injury. *(Courtesy Dr. Lisa Kohler, Summit County Medical Examiner, Akron, Ohio.)*

Burns from a steam iron often have a sharp, pointed margin from the tip of the instrument, whereas those from a curling iron are linear with the general width of approximately 1 cm and varying lengths. These types of burns are not exclusive to exposed skin surfaces (Figure 2-30). Another example of a burn not exclusive to skin surfaces is one caused by a caustic substance thrown into the eyes (see Figure 2-35). Immersion burns from hot water and scalds from throwing hot liquids are also observed (Figures 2-31 through 2-33). Burns may also be caused by a lighted cigarette (Figure 2-34).

Before cleaning and repairing the wound, carefully examine it for details such as length and depth of the wound, asymmetry of the wound, ragged or clean wound edges, accompanying abrasions or contusions at the site of the wound, and foreign bodies, such as wood splinters, glass shards, or debris in or around the wound. Document all findings.

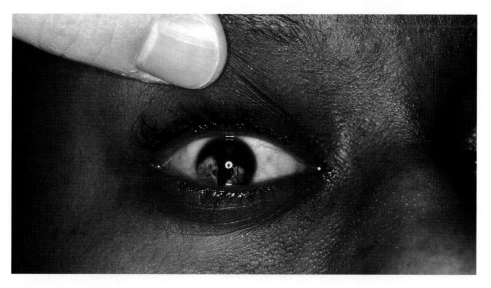

FIGURE 2-30 Burn caused by a curling iron. *(Courtesy Dr. David Effron, MetroHealth Medical Center, Cleveland, Ohio.)*

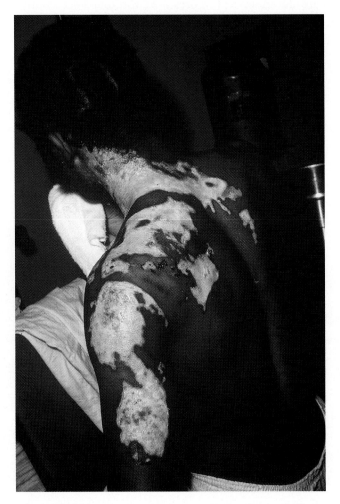

FIGURE 2-31   Burn scald from hot oatmeal. *(Courtesy Dr. David Effron, MetroHealth Medical Center, Cleveland, Ohio.)*

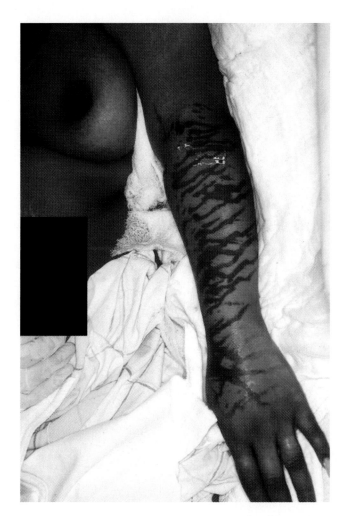

FIGURE 2-32   Burn assault. *(Courtesy Dr. David Effron, MetroHealth Medical Center, Cleveland, Ohio.)*

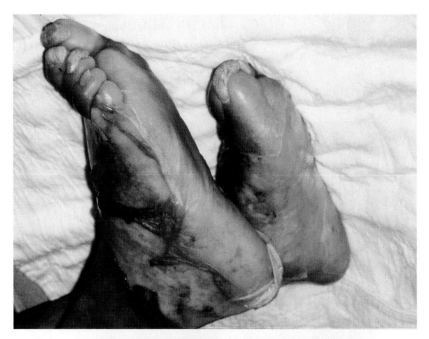

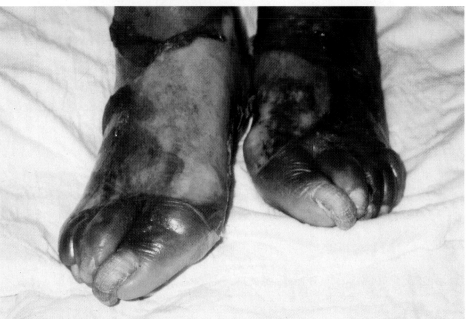

FIGURE 2-33   Burns to feet. *(Courtesy Dr. David Effron, MetroHealth Medical Center, Cleveland, Ohio.)*

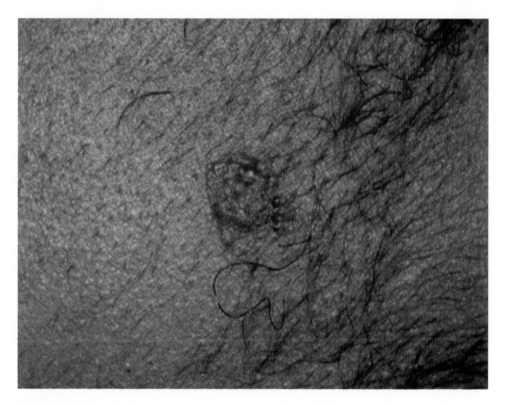

FIGURE 2-34   Healing cigarette burn. *(Courtesy The DOVE Program, Summa Health System, Akron, Ohio.)*

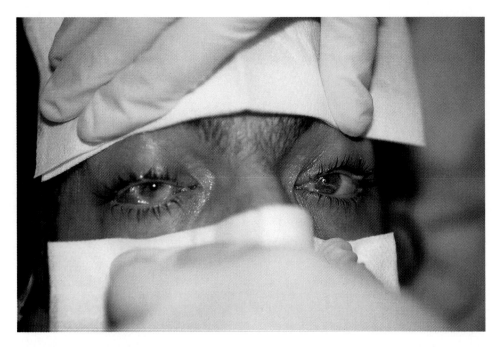

FIGURE 2-35 Lye burn to eye. *(Courtesy Dr. David Effron, MetroHealth Medical Center, Cleveland, Ohio.)*

Even in cases in which there has been no disclosure of domestic violence, certain types of injuries are red flags for physical abuse and should be explored further (Box 2-1).[2] Some injuries, such as cigarette burns, bite wounds, and some types of fractures, are fairly obvious. Others, however, such as impact bruising, abrasions and lacerations to hands and arms (defensive wounds) (Figures 2-36 through 2-38), traumatic alopecia, and fingertip patterned bruising, may be less obvious, especially for the clinician not used to screening for domestic violence. Having the patient undress fully and not limiting the examination to any one area of the body may help identify some of these types of injuries more easily and more consistently.

Box 2-1 *Common Injury Patterns in Domestic Violence*

- Slap marks from hands, with digits delineated
- Looped or flat contusions from belts or cords
- Contusions from fingertip pressure
- Scratches from fingernails
- Parallel contusions from contact with a linear object such as a baseball bat
- Contusions from shoe heels and soles
- Semicircular contusions or contused abrasions from bites

From Smock WS: The forensic aspect of caring for victims of domestic assault: identification of pattern injuries, *Physicians Violence-Free Soc Action Notes* 24:1-3, 1997.

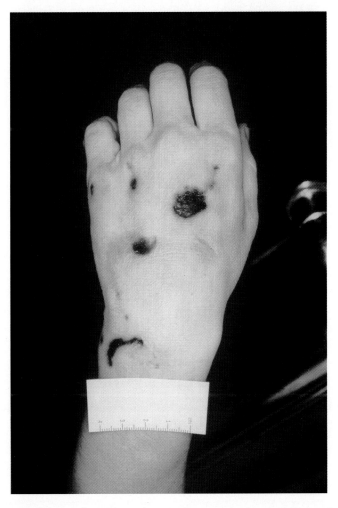

FIGURE 2-36 Defensive abrasions and contusions to the hand. *(Courtesy Dr. Lisa Kohler, Summit County Medical Examiner, Akron, Ohio.)*

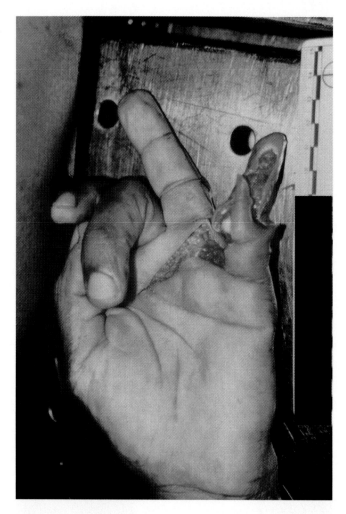

FIGURE 2-37 Incised wound to the hand as a result of a defensive posture. *(Courtesy Dr. Lisa Kohler, Summit County Medical Examiner, Akron, Ohio.)*

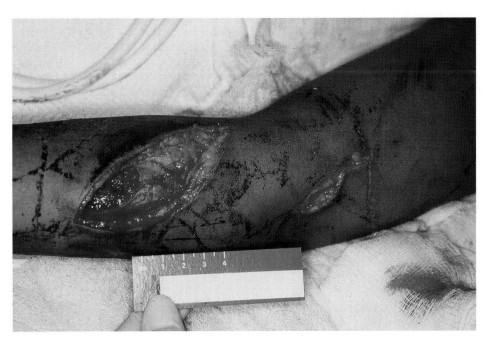

FIGURE 2-38 Defensive laceration on arm. *(Courtesy Dr. David Effron, MetroHealth Medical Center, Cleveland, Ohio.)*

SUMMARY AND CONCLUSION

Injury patterns and patterned injuries can provide vital clues regarding mechanism and force of injury. The presence of such injury must be carefully documented, using appropriate terminology and accompanying photographs and diagrams. Providing this type of detailed documentation ensures a visual record of the injury, long after the wounds heal. Although not every case of domestic violence is best served by law enforcement involvement, should the case enter the criminal justice arena, this documentation becomes especially useful if the victim recants his or her story or is unavailable for court testimony at a later date.

REFERENCES

1. Sheridan DJ: Treating survivors of intimate partner abuse: forensic identification and documentation. In Olshaker JS, Jackson MC, Smock WS, eds: *Forensic emergency medicine,* Philadelphia, 2001, Lippincott Williams & Wilkins.
2. Smock WS: Forensic emergency medicine. In Olshaker JS, Jackson MC, Smock WS, eds: *Forensic emergency medicine,* Philadelphia, 2001, Lippincott Williams & Wilkins.
3. Davis GJ: Pattern of injury: blunt and sharp, *Clin Lab Med* 18(1):339-350, 1998.
4. Zillmer DA: Domestic violence: the role of the orthopaedic surgeon in identification and treatment, *J Am Acad Orthop Surg* 8(2):91-96, 2000.
5. Brink O, Vesterby A, Jensen J: Pattern of injury due to interpersonal violence, *Injury* 29(9):705-709, 1998.
6. Shepherd JP and others: Pattern, severity and aetiology of injuries in victims of assault, *J Royal Soc Med* 83(2):75-78, 1990.
7. Strack GB, McClane G: *Documenting and prosecuting strangulation cases.* Presentation given June, 2002, Delaware County Prosecutor's Office, Delaware, OH.
8. Smock WS: The forensic aspect of caring for victims of domestic assault: identification of pattern injuries, *Physicians Violence-Free Soc Action Notes* 24:1-3, 1997.

3 APPROACH TO THE SERIOUS OR MULTIPLE TRAUMA PATIENT

S. Scott Polsky • Jenifer Markowitz • David Effron

Although many victims of domestic violence present with injuries that are not life-threatening, some injuries can have catastrophic consequences. It is the responsibility of the entire medical community to recognize such injuries and direct the patient to a surgeon schooled in trauma techniques. The American College of Surgeons, in its position statement on domestic violence, "recognizes that domestic violence is a major public health problem for children, intimate partners, and the elderly, with victims frequently needing surgical care." They go on to state that the treating physician is responsible "not only to care for the immediate injury and to reassure the patient, but also to identify and report potential threats to his or her safety, and to encourage an ongoing safety strategy."[1]

FORENSIC APPROACH TO PATIENT

Every domestic violence victim should be examined with the assumption that this information eventually will be used in a court of law. Evidence is much more difficult to obtain at a later date, so clinicians should approach the examination looking for, preserving, and documenting evidence of a crime at the moment the patient presents.

It is imperative that the patient's clothing is carefully examined for tears or holes. If the clothing must be cut off the patient, special care should be taken to leave these tears and holes intact. When cutting clothing off the victim, cut around tears and holes because these may serve to demonstrate the angle or distance from which force was initiated. Avoid cross-contamination of evidence (i.e., blood soaking through), and keep surfaces from touching each other. Dry evidence, such as hair or fibers, may be preserved in plastic bags or self-sealing envelopes. Any wet evidence, such as clothing, should be air-dried before packaging. If this is not possible, it should be collected in paper bags and air-dried immediately once in custody. See Chapter 4 for information regarding chain-of-custody issues.

Whenever possible, wounds should be observed and carefully documented before alteration (e.g., cleansing or suturing), and such alterations should be noted. Photographs are ideal, but diagrams and sketches with measurements also are useful. Some penetrating wounds, such as stab wounds, should be approximated then photographed before repair, to document the type of weapon used. Signed consent must be obtained before photographing any wound. When photographing an injury, a ruler or other standard object (e.g., a quarter) should be placed in the picture as a point of reference to show the size of the wound. Each wound should be photographed after obtaining a full-frame identification picture of the patient.[2] A 35-mm camera can be used and will produce the highest quality photographs. A new roll of film should be used for each patient. Use of this type of camera, however, depends on clinician skill. For the clinician unfamiliar with the use of a 35-mm camera, instant photography can be employed. It is often more convenient and more affordable and develops immediately, guaranteeing photographs that capture the images desired. If instant photography is used, the equipment must be adequate for capturing close-range shots. The basic Polaroid camera alone will be useful only for long-range shots. However, attachments are available in the Polaroid Spectra law enforcement kit that will allow midrange and close-range photography. Polaroid also makes an instant camera with macro capabilities—the SLR Macro 5; this camera is useful for magnifying wound detail not visible with standard instant photography.

Many clinicians are now employing digital photography, although some courts have challenged the admissibility of these photographs because of the ease in which they can be altered. If there is any question, clinicians should consult area law enforcement to determine preferred photography methods. Recommendations for enhancing admissibility of digital photos include preserving the original digital image on a hard drive or CD; preserving the original image alongside any altered version of that image should enhancement of the image be necessary; and maintaining meticulous chain of custody, including the name of the person who took the photograph, the time and date of the photograph, where and how the image was stored, and who had access to that photo.[3] Regardless of the manner in which the photo was taken, all photographs should be labeled with a minimum of the patient's name, hospital identification number, date, and name of the photographer. Photographs should include a full-frame identification photo, a midrange photo identifying the region of the body involved and a close-up photo to show the detail of the injury. The clinician must adhere to strict chain of custody with both undeveloped film and processed photographs until mounting them in the chart. Please refer to Besant-Matthews and Smock's excellent chapter on forensic photography in the emergency department in *Forensic Emergency Medicine* for further information.[4]

PHYSICAL EXAMINATION: THE PRIMARY SURVEY

All patients presenting with a history suggestive of significant trauma should have a primary survey. The approach is the same for both blunt and penetrating trauma. The focus of the primary survey is to identify and to prioritize and treat potential threats to life and limb. The American College of Surgeons in its text *Advanced Trauma Life Support (ATLS)*[5] describes this process as the *ABCDEs* of trauma care, as follows:

A = Airway
B = Breathing
C = Circulation including hemorrhage control
D = Disability or neurologic status
E = Exposure and Environmental control, meaning completely undress the patient to
      reveal all injuries but prevent hypothermia

In the traditional approach used in medicine, the practitioner gathers and analyzes as complete a set of data as possible before initiating treatment. However, in the care of the severe trauma patient, management of life-threatening conditions is initiated as they are discovered. Each potential life threat is identified and addressed in its order of importance to maximize the potential for survival. Resuscitation is simultaneous with assessment during the primary survey.

No patient will survive if he or she has airway compromise or cannot breathe. This is therefore the first priority. Control of the cervical spine is vital to prevent neurologic damage while the airway is secured.

Once the airway is secure, attention turns to the patient's circulation. Hypotension in the trauma patient should be treated as hypovolemia from blood loss until proven otherwise. A rapid, thready pulse is often a sign of hypovolemia. Ashen gray skin on the face and pale skin are often present with severe hypovolemia. Any external hemorrhage must be identified and controlled. Intravenous access is established, and blood samples are drawn for appropriate laboratory testing.

Disability assessment through a neurologic examination completes the primary survey. ATLS suggests using *AVPU* for assessment of level of consciousness, as follows[5]:

A = Alert
V = Verbal stimulus causes a response
P = Painful stimulus is required to cause a response
U = Unresponsive to stimulus

This system allows easy reproducibility among observers and does not require the use of terms that may be defined differently among observers.

Visualization is of paramount importance. When the patient is not completely disrobed and examined, significant injuries may be missed, with tragic consequences. It is also vital that the patient be kept warm. Resuscitation often entails large volumes of fluid replacement with solutions that are cooler than body temperature. The combination of exposure and fluid replacement can lead to hypothermia.

The major trauma patient requires monitoring multiple parameters that may include cardiac rhythm, arterial blood gases, carbon dioxide, continuous oxygenation via pulse oximetry, respirations, blood pressure, and temperature. X-ray examination that includes at least anteroposterior (AP) chest, AP pelvis, and lateral cervical spine films should be done early but must not interfere with the resuscitation process.

SECONDARY SURVEY AND HISTORY

The secondary survey includes an abbreviated history and a head-to-toe examination of the patient with a more detailed neurologic examination, including assessment using the Glasgow Coma Scale (GCS). Understanding the mechanism of injury helps to point to potential associated injury patterns. The concept of the secondary survey is to ensure identification of all injuries at this time.

The history may not be obtainable from a severely injured patient. Information from pre-hospital personnel and family can be extremely important. The model suggested by ATLS is called the *AMPLE* history[5]:

A = Allergies
M = Medications currently used
P = Past illnesses and Pregnancy
L = Last meal
E = Events and Environment related to the injury

The physical examination then proceeds from head to toe and includes the head, face, neck, cervical spine, chest, abdomen, perineum, rectum, and musculoskeletal and neurologic systems. As stated previously, care must be taken to identify all injuries. This includes more obvious injuries, such as those from blunt and penetrating trauma, and more subtle injuries, such as those resulting from strangulation. For a summary of signs and symptoms secondary to strangulation, please refer to Box 3-1.[6]

Box 3-1	*Signs and Symptoms of Strangulation Injury*

- Vocal changes
- Swallowing difficulties
- Difficulty breathing
- Mental status changes including combativeness and restlessness
- Involuntary urination and defecation
- Visible injuries, including patterned injuries to neck, including abrasions, contusions, and patterned redness
- Swelling of the neck secondary to internal bleeding, injury to underlying structures, and/or subcutaneous emphysema form a larynx fracture

Modified from Strack GB, McClane G: *Documenting and prosecuting strangulation cases.* Presentation given June, 2002, Delaware County Prosecutor's Office, Delaware, Ohio.

REFERENCES

1. American College of Surgeons, ST-32 statement on domestic violence: *Bull Am Coll Surgeons* 85(2), 2000.
2. Sheridan DJ: Treating survivors of intimate partner abuse: forensic identification and documentation. In Olshaker JS, Jackson MC, Smock WS, eds: *Forensic emergency medicine,* Philadelphia, 2001, Lippincott Williams & Wilkins.
3. Shaw C: Admissibility of digital photographic evidence: should it be any different than traditional photography? *NCPCA Update Newslett* 15(10), 2002.
4. Besant-Matthews PE, Smock WS: Forensic photography in the emergency department. In Olshaker JS, Jackson MC, Smock WS, eds: *Forensic emergency medicine,* Philadelphia, 2001, Lippincott Williams & Wilkins.
5. American College of Surgeons Committee on Trauma: *Advanced trauma life support student manual,* ed 6, Chicago, 1997, American College of Surgeons.
6. Strack GB, and McClane G: *Documenting and prosecuting strangulation cases.* Presentation given June, 2002 Delaware County Prosecutor's Office, Delaware, OH.

SUGGESTED READINGS

Pasqualone GA: Forensic RNs as photographers: documentation in the ED, *J Psychosoc Nurs* 34(10):47-51, 1996.
Stack LB and others: *Handbook of medical photography,* Philadelphia, 2001, Hanley & Belfus.
Staggs S: *Crime scene and evidence photographer's guide,* Temeula, Calif, 1997, Staggs Publishing.

4 PENETRATING INJURIES

Eileen F. Baker

FIREARMS VIOLENCE

Violence involving firearms accounted for 66% of all murders in the United States in 2001. Furthermore, during that same year, more than half a million violent crimes not resulting in death were committed with a firearm.[1] Nonfatal firearm-related injuries outnumber fatal injuries by 3 to 1.[2] An analysis of all shootings in three U.S. cities over 18 months found that one third of shootings occurred in or near a residence. Of these, two thirds took place in the home of the victim and only 9% were unintentional. Suicide accounted for 19% of residential shootings, and assaults accounted for 70%.[3] According to a review of national data related to murder-suicides in the United States, almost 95% of these crimes involve firearms. In the first 6 months of 2001, Florida, California, and Texas led the nation in murder-suicide events with 35, 29, and 29, respectively.[4]

HANDGUNS

Handguns constitute about one third of the nation's firearms, yet account for 70% to 90% of fatal firearm injuries. They are five times more likely to be kept loaded than long guns are.[5] Handguns are firearms that can be held and fired with one hand. Bullets are metal projectiles, usually made of lead or steel, in various shapes (Figure 4-1). Bullets may be covered with a jacket of metal or copper. Some projectiles are designed to lose their energy inside the target (so-called "safety slugs," often used by law enforcement agencies). These cause greater destruction within the target mass but are less likely to pass through the target or to ricochet. The size of a handgun is determined by the diameter of the cartridge it fires. This is measured in millimeters or hundredths of an inch and is known as the *caliber*. Some common diameters include 9-mm, .22 (22-caliber), and .38 (38-caliber).

BALLISTICS

Not only the bullet is fired from the gun, but also other substances such as gases, gunshot residue (GSR), incompletely burned pieces of gunpowder, and metal fragments are issued forth. Each of these may provide forensic clues and should be preserved as evidence. Presence

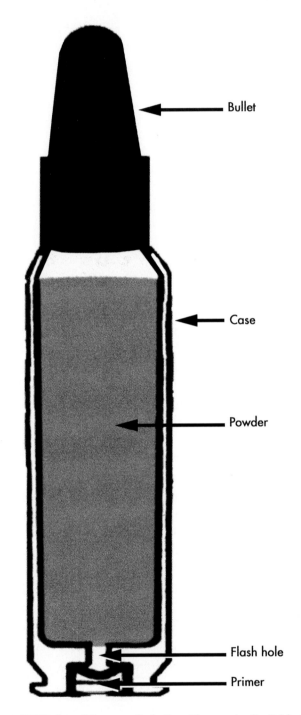

FIGURE 4-1   Diagram of a bullet. *(Courtesy Analise Polsky.)*

or absence of such indicators may provide clues as to the range of fire (the distance from the muzzle of gun to the victim) and help identify entrance and exit wounds. Hence, close attention to these details and documentation, through written description, photographs, and collection of evidence, is essential.

ENTRANCE WOUNDS, EXIT WOUNDS, AND CLUES TO RANGE OF FIRE

Some common assumptions are that entrance wounds are small, exit wounds are large, and the caliber of the bullet correlates with the size of the wound. In fact, however, entrance wound size is not related to the caliber of the bullet. Entrance wounds over elastic tissue can contract around the wound and have a diameter measuring less than the caliber of the bullet. Furthermore, exit wound size is determined by the amount of energy possessed by the bullet as it exits the skin, as well as the bullet's size and configuration. The exit wound is not necessarily larger than the entrance wound.

Entrance wounds can be categorized as contact, near contact/close range, intermediate/medium range, and indeterminate/distant range. Distant-range wounds are of 2 feet or more. Only the bullet makes contact with the skin, and no tattooing or GSR deposition is seen. As the bullet penetrates, the skin is indented, leaving an abrasion collar. The abrasion collar is an abraded area of tissue surrounding the wound (typically an entrance wound). The width may vary with the angle of impact. On palms or soles, however, no abrasion collar is noted and the wound appears slit-like (Figures 4-2 and 4-3). Intermediate-range wounds (6 inches to 2 feet) are characterized by tattooing. Tattooing results from contact with partially burned or unburned grains of gunpowder. This injury is caused by abrasions by the grains of gunpowder striking the skin. This cannot be wiped away, unlike GSR.

Near-contact wounds (less than 6 inches) demonstrate the maximum range at which GSR is deposited on the wound or clothing. GSR wipes off of the skin, unlike tattooing.

In contact wounds, the barrel is in contact with the skin or clothing when discharged. These may vary in appearance from a small hole with seared, blackened edges to gaping, stellate wounds. Large wounds, caused by expansion of the skin with gases, are often misinterpreted as exit wounds. With tight-contact wounds, hot gases, metal fragments, gunpowder, and flame all are discharged into the wound. The skin stretches with expansion of gases, resulting in triangular-shaped tears. The base of the triangle overlies the entrance of the wound (Figure 4-4). In tight-contact wounds over softer tissue, the expanding skin is forced back against the muzzle, resulting in a patterned abrasion (muzzle contusion) (Figure 4-5).

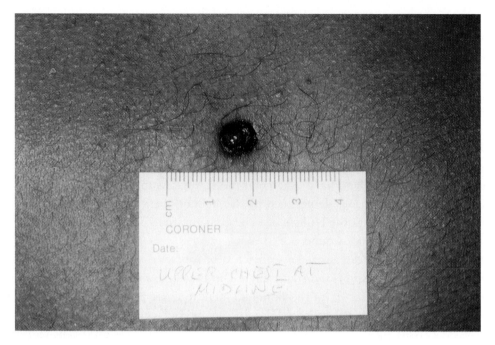

FIGURE 4-2 Distant chest entry wound. *(Courtesy Dr. Lisa Kohler, Summit County Medical Examiner's Office, Akron, Ohio.)*

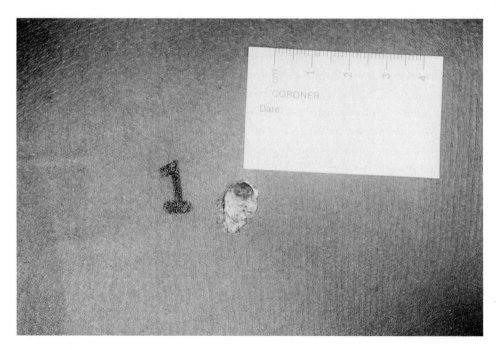

FIGURE 4-3 Distant angled chest entry wound. *(Courtesy Dr. Lisa Kohler, Summit County Medical Examiner's Office, Akron, Ohio.)*

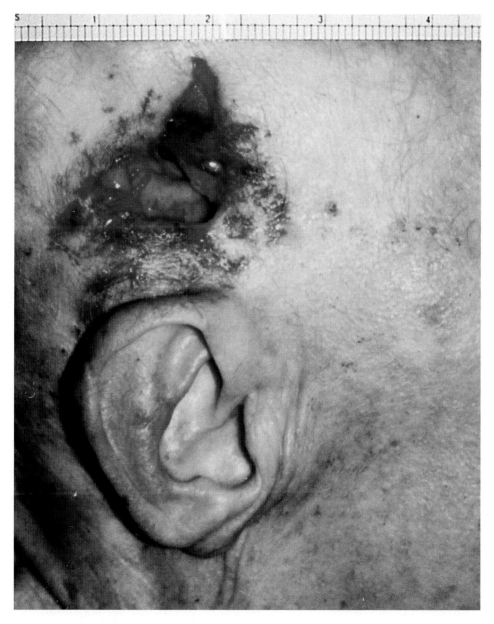

FIGURE 4-4 Tight contact gunshot wound to the head. Note the triangular-shaped tear resulting from expansion of hot gases. *(Courtesy Dr. Lisa Kohler, Summit County Medical Examiner's Office, Akron, Ohio.)*

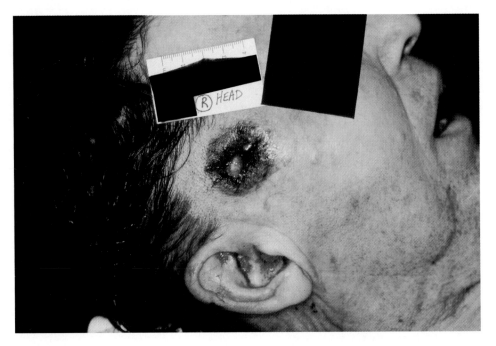

FIGURE 4-5   Tight contact entry wound to head with muzzle contusion. *(Courtesy Dr. Lisa Kohler, Summit County Medical Examiner's Office, Akron, Ohio.)*

Exit wounds are the result of the bullet (and bone) pushing and stretching the skin from inside out. Skin edges are typically everted, with sharp, irregular margins. Generally, no abrasion collars or GSR is seen. Tattooing is never observed.

GRAZE WOUNDS

Graze wounds result from tangential contact with a passing bullet. The direction of the bullet can be determined through careful examination of the wound. As the bullet passes along the skin, skin tags are formed on the lateral wound margins. The base of the skin tags point toward the weapon and away from the direction of bullet travel (Figures 4-6 and 4-7).

SHOTGUNS

Shotgun shells traditionally consist of a brass head, a primer, powder, wads generally made of paper or cardboard, and lead shot. More recently, shells have been made of polyethylene, color-coded by gauge to prevent using the wrong gauge ammunition in a given weapon. The tube length of the shell may vary with the type of ammunition (Figure 4-8).

As the shot issues forth from the shotgun barrel, it spreads. The pattern of spread can vary with the degree of *choke* in the barrel. The barrel of the shotgun can be removed so that barrels of different choke can be inserted. At times, the shotgun barrel may be "sawed off," making the weapon more concealable. At distances of 21 feet or less, the size of the shot pattern is largely unaffected until the barrel has been sawed off to less than 9 inches.

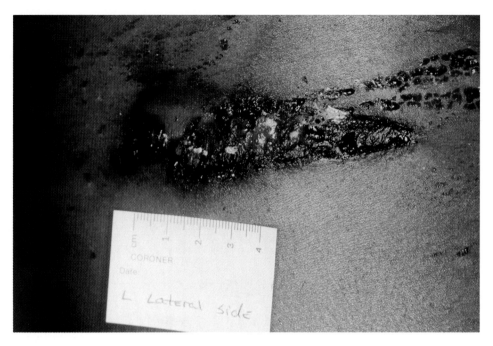

FIGURE 4-6   Graze wounds. *(Courtesy Dr. Lisa Kohler, Summit County Medical Examiner's Office, Akron, Ohio.)*

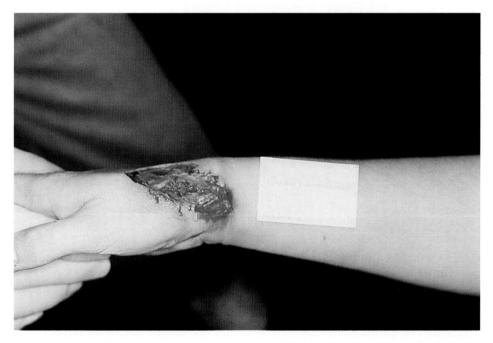

FIGURE 4-7   Graze wounds. *(Courtesy Dr. Lisa Kohler, Summit County Medical Examiner's Office, Akron, Ohio.)*

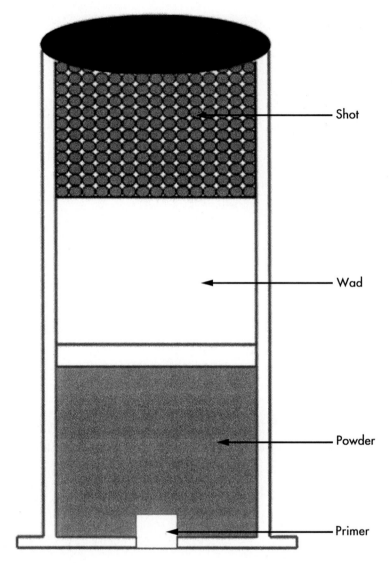

FIGURE 4-8 Diagram of shotgun shell cross section. *(Courtesy Analise Polsky.)*

Shot

Shot may be composed of lead, lead with antimony, or lead plated with copper or nickel. Shot composed of steel, bismuth, or tungsten is commonly used in migratory bird hunting. Birdshot is used for hunting birds and ranges from 12-gauge (0.05 inches in diameter) to BBs (0.18 inches in diameter). BB shot is not the same as commonly known "BBs" used in air rifles (BB guns). Buckshot ranges from 0.24 to 0.36 inches in diameter and is numbered based on the number of pellets in the shell, rather than the weight of the charge or gauge (Figure 4-9).

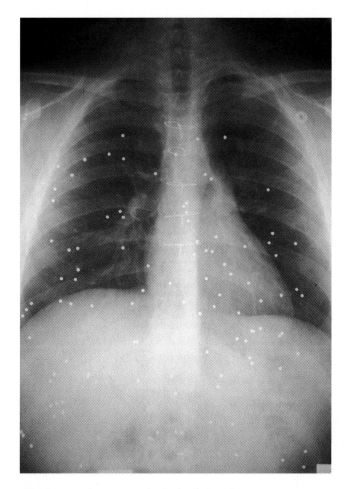

FIGURE 4-9   Chest x-ray showing multiple buckshot fragments. *(Courtesy Dr. David Effron, MetroHealth Medical Center, Cleveland, Ohio.)*

Shotgun Slugs and Slug Wounds

Wounds caused by shotgun slugs are typically round and approximately the same diameter as the slug. An abrasion collar may be present. Wads from the slug produce circular or oval imprints at close range. Slugs are designed to "pancake" or flatten within a target or may break into pieces.

Shotgun Wounds

The shotgun at close range is the most destructive of all small arms. The number of pellets entering the body, their location, organ damage, and tissue destruction determine the lethality of the shotgun wound.

Because shot disperses with greater distance, the farther from the target, the fewer pellets that strike the target. Also, the velocity of the pellets drops off quickly, so damage is minimal at distant range and may have insufficient velocity even to penetrate skin.

Contact wounds of the head are obviously devastating, because the cranium is generally fractured, the brain is shredded, and the scalp is extensively lacerated. The shot pellets not only induce direct tissue injury but also cause pressure waves that may increase the destruction of the shot, while gases from combustion expand rapidly and add to these pressure waves. Shattering of the skull results (Figure 4-10).

Most contact shotgun wounds to the head are a result of suicide. Intraoral shotgun wounds result in deposition of GSR on the palate, tongue, and lips. Lacerations of the lips or naso-labial folds result from the expansion of gases within the mouth.

Contact wounds of the trunk are typically circular, with a diameter approximating that of the bore of the weapon. Because the gases disperse within the body cavity, skin tears are not seen. Hard contact wounds may cause searing and blackening by hot gases, but no GSR is found. Patterned abrasions from the muzzle of the weapon can be encountered, and abrasion collars can be found (Figure 4-11).

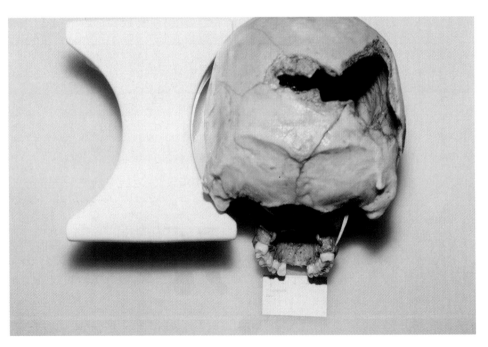

FIGURE 4-10   Gunshot wound to the skull. (*Courtesy Dr. Lisa Kohler, Summit County Medical Examiner's Office, Akron, Ohio.*)

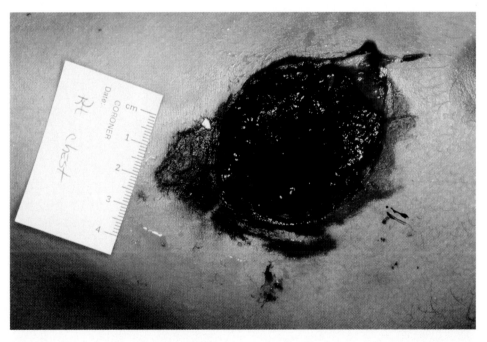

FIGURE 4-11   Contact shotgun wound with muzzle abrasion. *(Courtesy Dr. Lisa Kohler, Summit County Medical Examiner's Office, Akron, Ohio.)*

SHARP-FORCE INJURIES

Terminology is key in describing sharp-force injuries. Two types of such injuries are recognized: *incised* and *stab* wounds. Incised wounds are longer than they are deep (Figure 4-12). Stab wounds are puncture wounds that are deeper than they are wide. Sharp weapons do not impart "lacerations" per se, but "incisional lacerations." A "laceration" results from blunt-force trauma, such as when one's forehead strikes a steering wheel. Bridging of tissue is evident. Sharp-force injuries impart clean wound margins, unlike the abraded edges seen in blunt-force trauma.

Examination of a knife's "anatomy" explains the types of wound patterns found. The handle allows the operator to grip the weapon. A single-edged knife blade has both a sharp edge and a dull edge, which render characteristic wound patterns. Double-edged knife blades bear two sharp edges. Both double- and single-edged blades have a hilt, where the proximal end of the blade meets the handle. If plunged deeply into the body, a characteristic *hilt mark* may be seen (Figure 4-13).

Patterns resulting from serrated versus sharp blades may be determined only if the blade was drawn across the skin during its insertion or withdrawal. Because these characteristic marks may not be found, one may not always recover evidence that a serrated blade was used.

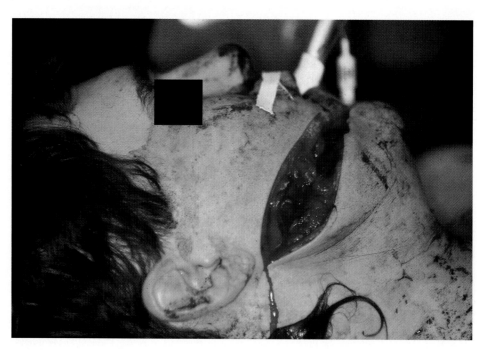

FIGURE 4-12 Photograph of a face laceration. *(Courtesy Dr. David Effron, MetroHealth Medical Center, Cleveland, Ohio.)*

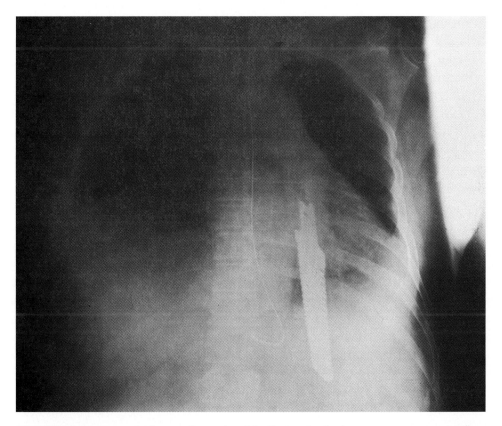

FIGURE 4-13 Lateral chest radiograph of knife in the back. *(Courtesy Dr. David Effron, MetroHealth Medical Center, Cleveland, Ohio.)*

Self-Inflicted Sharp-Force Injuries

Self-inflicted wounds should be suspected in patients who present with multiple incised wounds, especially those of varying depth. So-called "hesitation marks" are the result of repeated, shallow incisions to the skin during which the patient "works up the nerve" to injure himself (Figure 4-14). Such wounds are common on the neck, wrists, chest, and face. All such patients should receive psychiatric evaluation for depression or other disorder.

FORENSIC EVIDENCE

The key to building a strong forensic case hinges on proper evidence collection and preservation. Forensic evidence includes photographs, clothing, and evidence on the hands of the victim. Such evidence may serve to identify a suspect, prove an element of a crime, or prove the theory of the case. Evidence can be compromised in a number of ways. Failure to recognize evidence, improper storage, and failure to maintain chain of custody are all too common.

GSR, soft lead, and lubricant (also known as *bullet wipe*) may be found on clothing overlying the entrance wound or on the wound itself around the abrasion collar. This appears as a gray rim or streak. Hence, any object that comes between the muzzle and the wound that prevents deposition of GSR, tattooing, or residues on the skin can be important evidence. These are termed *intermediate objects*. When such an object is an article of clothing, do not destroy the bullet hole. When cutting clothing off the victim, cut around bullet holes because these may serve to demonstrate the angle or distance from which the weapon was fired. Avoid cross-contamination of evidence (i.e., blood soaking through), and keep surfaces from touching each other. Dry evidence, such as hair or fibers, may be preserved in plastic bags or self-adhesive envelopes. Any wet evidence should be air-dried immediately and collected in paper bags. If drying is not possible before packaging, jelly roll the wet evidence in paper, a sheet, or a pillowcase before packaging to prevent cross contamination of trace evidence or minimization of osmosis. Once in custody, all items should be removed from packaging and air-dried immediately. The material for the "jelly roll" should also be dried and retained.

As noted earlier, whenever possible, wounds should be observed and findings documented before any alteration such as cleansing; any alteration should be documented as well. Photographs are ideal, but diagrams and sketches with measurements also are useful. It is best for medical personnel to avoid altering the appearance of wounds during medical intervention. For example, thoracostomy tubes should not be placed through wounds. When making a thoracotomy incision, physicians should avoid the temptation to "connect the dots" and should instead make a clean incision that avoids any chest wounds, wherever possible.

Bullets recovered from the victim should be handled with care. Again, metal instruments should not be used, to avoid introducing stray marks onto the bullet. Clothing may also be found in the wound, having been driven in by the bullet. Thus preservation of this evidence recovered from the wound, as well as the clothing of victim, is important.[6]

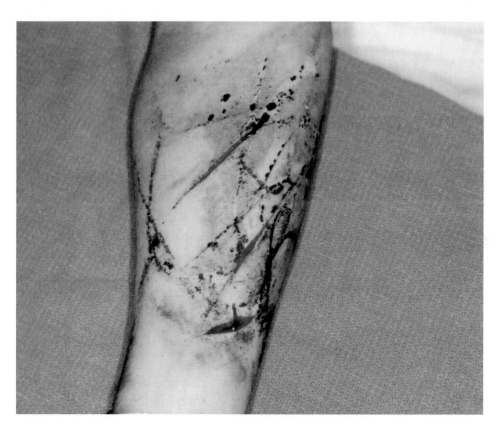

FIGURE 4-14 Hesitation marks as seen in patient-inflicted slicing wounds. *(Courtesy Jill Bunnell, RNc, FNE, The DOVE Program, Summa Health System, Akron, Ohio.)*

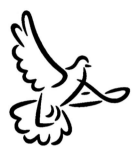

**DOVE PROGRAM
FORENSIC LAB
CHAIN OF CUSTODY FORM**

Date: _____

Subject's Name: _____

Address: _____

City: _____ State: _____ Zip: _____

Social Security Number: _____ DOB: _____ Sex: _____

Incident Report Number: _____

Case Number: _____

Charges: _____

Samples Obtained By: _____

Type of Sample(s) Obtained: _____

Place Obtained: _____

Date and Time Obtained: _____

Collection Witnessed by Officer/Detective: _____

Sample Submitted By: _____

Received From	Received By	Date	Time

Chain of Custody Form

FIGURE 4-15   Chain of custody form. *(Courtesy The DOVE Program, Summa Health System, Akron, Ohio.)*

Table 4-1 *Evidence Collection Summary*	
OBSERVATION	ACTION
Penetrating injury	Avoid placing tubes/drains in wounds.
	Avoid making surgical incisions through wounds.
	Photograph/document before and after cleansing.
	Photograph/document before and after reapproximation.
Bullet wound	Photograph/document before and after cleansing.
GSR	Photograph/document.
	Sample for firearms residue test.
Tattooing/stippling	Photograph/document.
Abrasion collar	Photograph/document.
Muzzle contusion	Photograph/document.
Bullet	Collect carefully; avoid using metal instruments or storage on metal trays.
Incised wound	Photograph/document before and after cleansing.
	Photograph/document before and after reapproximation.
Damaged clothing	Cut around (*not through*) bullet holes, incisions, and tears.
Clothing or other items	Maintain chain of custody.
Damp/wet clothes	Store in paper bags; alert law enforcement.
Dry clothes	Store in paper bags.
Dry items (hair/fiber)	Store in self-adhesive envelope, paper or plastic bag.

GSR, Gunshot residue.

THE CHAIN OF CUSTODY

The chain of custody is a method of obtaining, transporting, and storing evidence that demonstrates proof that evidence collected at the crime scene or from the patient is the same as that being presented in court (Figure 4-15). Proper handling and storage of evidence, as just described, is key. Aside from plastic and paper bags, plastic jars or vials, tamper-resistant tape, chain-of-custody forms, labels, and tags are all essential components of evidence collection (Table 4-1). Furthermore, documentation of their collection, transport, and transfer from person to person is of utmost importance.

REFERENCES

1. Rennison C: *Criminal victimization 2001,* Washington, DC, 2002, Bureau of Justice Statistics.
2. Cherry D and others: Trends in nonfatal and fatal firearm-related injury rates in the United States, 1985-1995, *Ann Emerg Med* 32(1):51-59, 1998.
3. Kellermann AL and others: Injuries and deaths due to firearms in the home, *J Trauma* 45(2):263-267, 1998.
4. Violence Policy Center: *American roulette: the untold story of murder-suicide in the United States,* Washington, DC, 2002, Violence Policy Center.
5. Powell KE and others: State estimates of household exposure to firearms, loaded firearms, and handguns, 1991 through 1995, *Am J Public Health* 88(6):969-972, 1998.
6. DiMaio VJ: *Gunshot wounds,* ed 2, Boca Raton, Fla, 1999, CRC Press.

5 ORAL AND FACIAL INJURIES

Michael Powers • James Connors

Domestic violence frequently results in facial injuries. Berrios and Grady[1] found that 68% of women diagnosed as abused sustained injury to the facial area. In cases of domestic violence involving children, trauma to the head and associated areas occurs approximately 50% of the time.[2]

Because facial injuries are common occurrences, it is imperative that clinicians involved in the initial presentation of these patients be well versed in the assessment and management of oral and facial trauma. This section is designed to be a guide for the nonspecialist to offer abused patients the best chance for appropriate care of their oral, dental, and facial injuries.

STEP-WISE EXAMINATION

Extra-Oral Examination

Initial clinical examinations should be methodical and are commonly approached beginning with the extra-oral examination as follows:

1. Soft tissues
2. Nerves
3. Skeleton

Soft Tissue

Examination of facial soft tissues should include cleansing of abrasions and lacerations and probing of the latter for foreign bodies. Periorbital lacerations, subconjunctival hemorrhage, and blood in the anterior chamber (Figures 5-1 and 5-2) should prompt an ophthalmologic consult, because injury to the globe may have occurred. Similarly, a neurosurgical consult should be obtained after examination of the external auditory meatus and nares if cerebrospinal fluid (CSF) otorrhea or rhinorrhea is found. Bilateral ecchymosis around or behind the ears (Battle sign) (Figure 5-3) associated with head trauma can result from violation of the cranium via basilar skull, ethmoid, sphenoid, and frontal bone fractures (Figure 5-4). Ecchymosis around both eyes (raccoon eyes) is also associated with basilar skull fractures (Figure 5-5).

Text continued on page 86

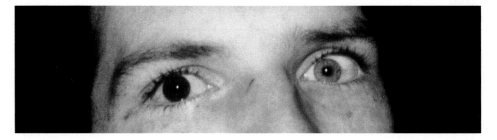

FIGURE 5-1   Blood in the anterior chamber. *(Courtesy Dr. Scott Polsky, Summa Health System, Akron, Ohio.)*

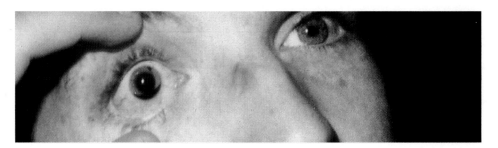

FIGURE 5-2   Hyphema. *(Courtesy Dr. Scott Polsky, Summa Health System, Akron, Ohio.)*

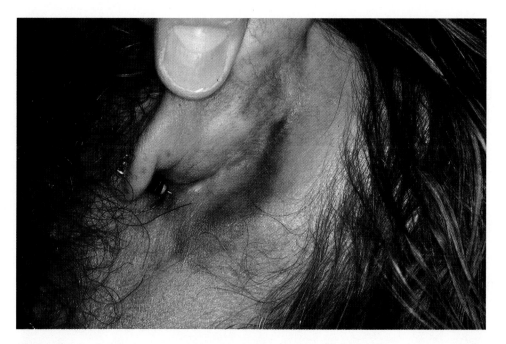

FIGURE 5-3   Battle sign. *(Courtesy Dr. David Effron, MetroHealth Medical Center, Cleveland, Ohio.)*

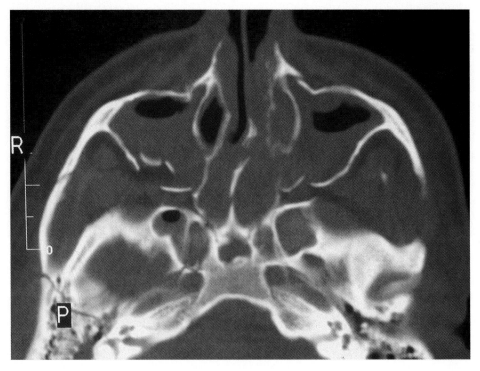

FIGURE 5-4   Orbital and basilar skull fractures. *(Courtesy Dr. David Effron, MetroHealth Medical Center, Cleveland, Ohio.)*

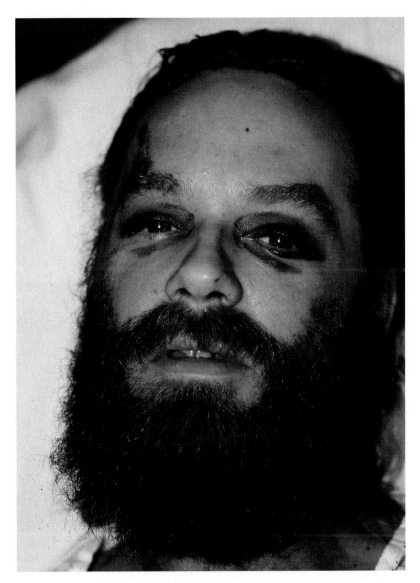

FIGURE 5-5   Raccoon sign. *(Courtesy Dr. David Effron, MetroHealth Medical Center, Cleveland, Ohio.)*

During the nasal examination, the septum should be evaluated for a possible hematoma. If found, it should be drained to prevent septal necrosis and perforation (Figures 5-6 and 5-7).

Nerves

The facial nerve (cranial nerve VII) controls the muscles of facial expression and is often damaged by lacerating injuries to the face. The clinician should ask the patient to make the following facial expressions:

1. Smile
2. Frown
3. Raise eyebrows
4. Close eyes tightly
5. Pucker lips and inflate cheeks

Damage to a branch of the facial nerve will manifest as a weakness of the muscles supplied by that branch and result in an asymmetry of movement. Any such weaknesses must be documented and requires consultation by an appropriate specialist.

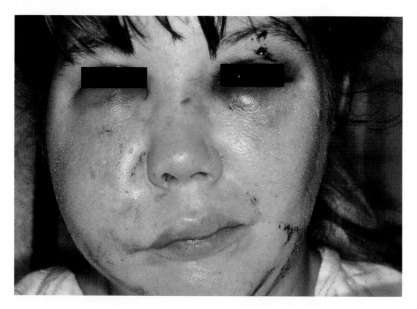

FIGURE 5-6 Nasoorbital fracture. (*Courtesy Dr. David Effron, MetroHealth Medical Center, Cleveland, Ohio.*)

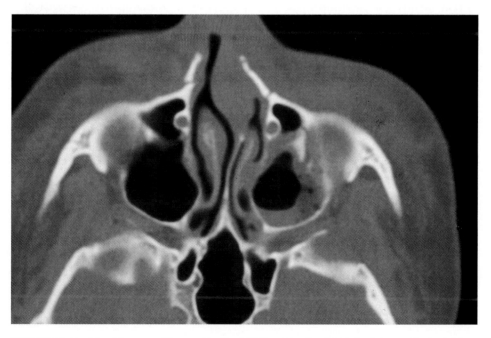

FIGURE 5-7   Nasal fracture. *(Courtesy Dr. David Effron, MetroHealth Medical Center, Cleveland, Ohio.)*

The infraorbital nerve provides sensation to the anterior mid-face. It is usually injured in orbital floor blowout fractures (Figures 5-8 and 5-9) and infraorbital rim fractures (Figure 5-10). Decreased sensation over areas supplied by this nerve should be documented.

The optic nerve is termed *special sensory* in nature and is responsible for vision. It can be injured intracranially or by compression by a fracture of the optic foramen as it passes through. Blindness or loss of light reflexes should prompt immediate neurosurgical and ophthalmologic evaluation.

The oculomotor nerve, among other functions, controls pupillary movement. Damage to this nerve is primarily via increased intracranial pressure and results in unequal or dilated pupils. Anisocoria (unequal pupils) in the presence of altered level of consciousness (LOC) is an ominous finding and should result in an immediate neurosurgical consult. If anisocoria is found with a normal LOC, direct injury to the eye is the likely cause and an urgent ophthalmologic consult is warranted.

Injury to the abducens nerve is also most commonly central in origin and results in lateral rectus paralysis on lateral gaze. The affected eye is therefore unable to move laterally (Figure 5-11). The olfactory nerve conveys the sense of smell and is commonly injured in mid-face fractures that involve the cribriform plate. This results in anosmia (loss of the sense of smell).

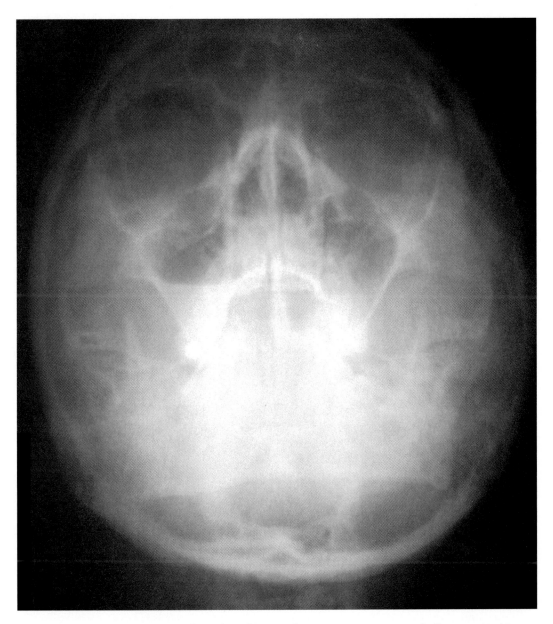

FIGURE 5-8   Radiograph of an orbital blowout fracture. *(Courtesy Dr. David Effron, MetroHealth Medical Center, Cleveland, Ohio.)*

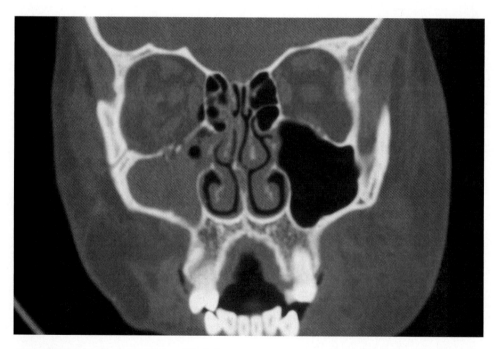

FIGURE 5-9 CT image of an orbital fracture. *(Courtesy Dr. David Effron, MetroHealth Medical Center, Cleveland, Ohio.)*

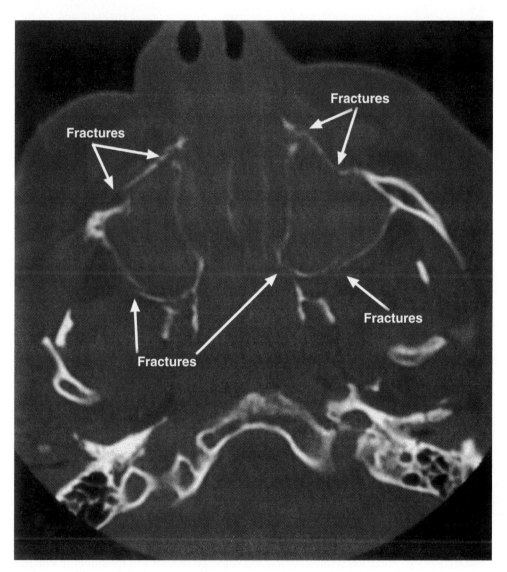

FIGURE 5-10   CT scan with multiple facial fractures. *(Courtesy Trauma Division, Summa Health System, Akron, Ohio.)*

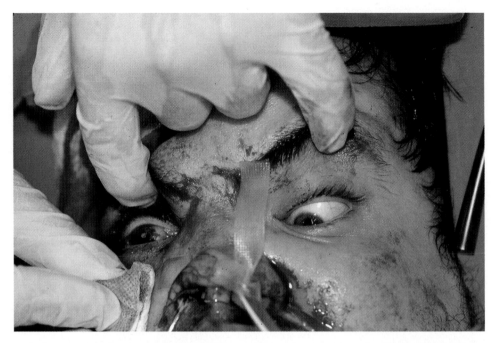

FIGURE 5-11 Photograph of an orbital fracture gaze. *(Courtesy Dr. David Effron, MetroHealth Medical Center, Cleveland, Ohio.)*

Skeleton

Because the mandible will be examined as part of the intraoral examination, attention can now be turned to the mid-face—specifically the maxilla and zygoma. The presence of the following are clues to the clinician that suggest the probability of a maxillary fracture:

- Intra-oral maxillary buccal vestibule swelling and ecchymosis
- Sagittal palatal lacerations
- Vertical maxillary gingival lacerations
- Mobile groups of maxillary teeth
- Malocclusion of teeth in the absence of detectable mandibular damage detected during the intra-oral portion of the examination

The nasofrontal suture region should be grasped with the thumb and forefinger of one hand, while the inferior maxilla in the region of the anterior teeth is grasped with the other. The maxilla is then torqued in all three planes. Movement of the lower maxilla without motion at the nasofrontal suture is indicative of a Le Fort I fracture. Concomitant motion about the nasofrontal suture in the absence of motion about the lateral orbital rims indicates a Le Fort II fracture, whereas a Le Fort III fracture will include motion at the lateral orbital rims (Table 5-1) (Figures 5-12 and 5-13). Blood in the sinuses shown on computed tomography (CT) is an indicator of

Table 5-1 *Clinical Signs and Symptoms of Mandibular Facial Fractures*

FRACTURE	CONDYLE	SUBCONDYLAR	CORONOID	RAMUS	ANGLE	BODY	SYMPHYSIS	ALVEOLAR	FLAIL MANDIBLE	BILATERAL EDENTULOUS BODY
Airway obstruction	−	−	−	−	−	−	−	−	+	+
Asymmetry, facial	+	+	−	+	+	+	−	−	+	−
Crepitus	−	−	−	+	+	+	+	−	+	+
Deviation of mandibular opening	+	+	+	−	−	−	−	−	±	−
Ecchymosis, buccal vestibule	−	−	−	−	±	+	±	±	±	−
Ecchymosis, floor of mouth	−	−	−	−	−	+	+	±	+	+
Lengthening of face	±	±	−	−	−	±	−	−	±	+
Limitation of opening, trismus	+	+	+	+	+	+	+	−	+	+
Malocclusion	±	±	+	±	±	±	±	+	+	−
Mobility of teeth	−	−	−	−	±	±	±	+	±	−
Paresthesia, lower lip	−	−	−	±	±	±	−	−	−	+

+ = Consistent clinical finding; ± = possible finding; − = no clinical finding.
From Gerlock A.J. Jr, Sinn D.P., *Clinical and radiographic interpretation of facial fractures,* Boston, 1981, Little, Brown.

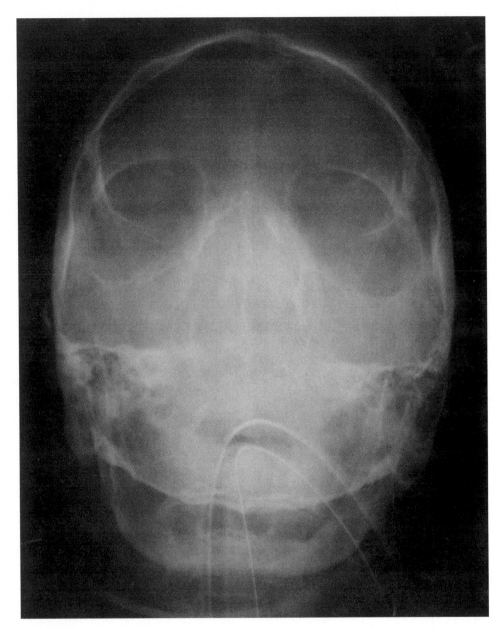

FIGURE 5-12 Posterior-anterior and lateral radiographs showing multiple facial fractures. *(Courtesy Trauma Division, Summa Health System, Akron, Ohio.)*

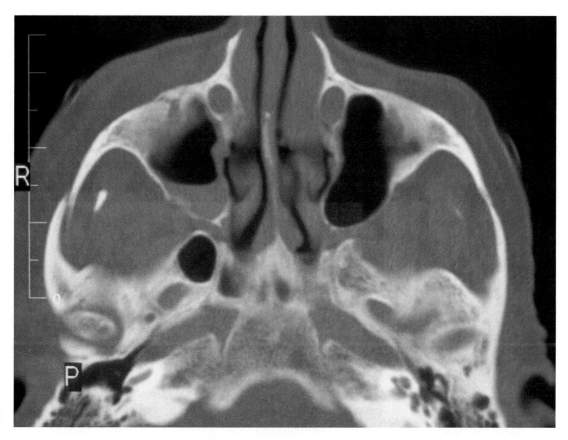

FIGURE 5-13   Facial CT demonstrating anterior and posterior orbital fractures and right zygoma fracture. *(Courtesy Dr. David Effron, MetroHealth Medical Center, Cleveland, Ohio.)*

facial fractures (Figure 5-14). One can now palpate the orbital rims for step-offs and the zygomatic arches for deformity. The arches can also be evaluated visually; this is best done by standing behind the head of the bed to gauge projection and symmetry of the patient's cheeks (Figures 5-15 and 5-16). Keep in mind that numbness about the rims and arches is a common finding with fractures in this area. It is also of note that visual disturbances can occur as a result of lateral canthal displacement in these injuries and by displacement of the orbital contents in orbital floor fractures. Thus it is appropriate to recheck visual acuity and extraocular muscle function at this time, and any abnormalities must be noted.

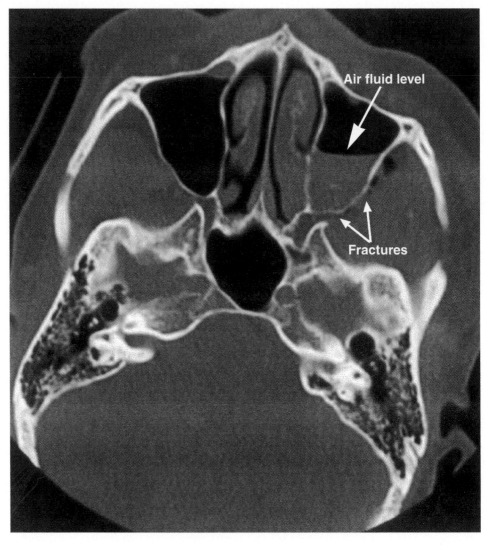

FIGURE 5-14   CT scan showing blood in the maxillary sinus from a facial fracture. *(Courtesy Trauma Division, Summa Health System, Akron, Ohio.)*

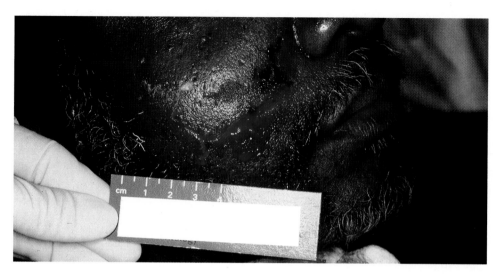

FIGURE 5-15 Photograph of a face bottle laceration zygoma fracture. *(Courtesy Dr. David Effron, MetroHealth Medical Center, Cleveland, Ohio.)*

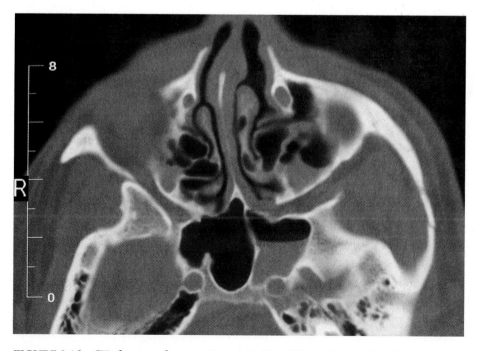

FIGURE 5-16 CT of zygoma fracture. *(Couresty Dr. David Effron, MetroHealth Medical Center, Cleveland, Ohio.)*

The last parts to be evaluated are the nasal–orbital–ethmoid suture complex and nose. The nasal bridge is examined for saddle deformity or deviation and is palpated for mobility. Damage to the nasoorbital–ethmoid complex typically results in an increase in medial intercanthal distance to a total greater than 32 mm, with a rounding of the normal acute angle of the canthus. This happens when the medial canthal ligaments are avulsed from their attachments in nasoorbital–ethmoid fractures.

Intra-Oral Examination

After completion of all parts of the extra-oral examination, the intra-oral examination is performed in a similarly strict manner, as follows:

1. Soft tissues
2. Nerves
3. Skeleton
4. Dentition

Intra-Oral Soft Tissue

The oral soft tissue examination begins with examination of the tongue, which is frequently lacerated (Figure 5-17). Bleeding should be controlled and wounds probed for foreign bodies such as tooth fragments. The floor of the mouth, gingiva, palate, buccal mucosa, and lips can then be examined in that order. Special attention should be paid to any oral swelling or ecchymosis or vertical tears of the gingiva or hard palate, because these are commonly associated with underlying fractures of the maxilla, mandible, or alveolus.

Nerves

After the soft tissue is thoroughly examined, attention should be turned to two nerves that are frequently affected:

- Injury to the *lingual nerve* results in anesthesia, paresthesia, and/or loss of taste to the anterior two thirds of the tongue on the affected side.
- Injury to the *inferior alveolar nerve* is usually the result of a fractured mandible and presents as numbness of the lower lip on the side of the fracture.

Skeleton

This portion of the oral examination is begun with examination of the mandible. It is helpful to know the mechanism of injury, because this can help pinpoint areas of potential fracture. For example, a blow with a fist to the left side of the face by a right-handed assailant very commonly results in right parasymphysis and left-angle mandibular fractures (Figures 5-18 and 5-19), whereas a direct blow to the chin frequently results in bilateral subcondylar fractures. The mandible is examined intra-orally and extra-orally through visualization and palpation. Edema, ecchymosis, crepitation, pain to palpation, and "steps" in the bony contour of the inferior border or the row of teeth of the lower jaw (Figures 5-20 and 5-21) all indicate

Text continued on page 103

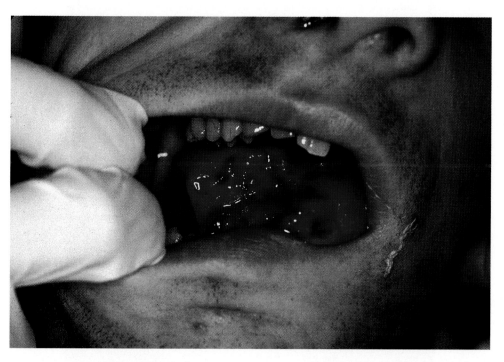

FIGURE 5-17 Photograph of a bitten tongue. *(Courtesy Dr. David Effron, MetroHealth Medical Center, Cleveland, Ohio.)*

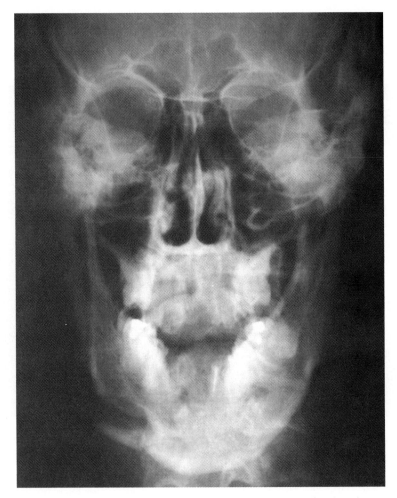

FIGURE 5-18 Radiograph of a mandible fracture. *(Courtesy Dr. David Effron, MetroHealth Medical Center, Cleveland, Ohio.)*

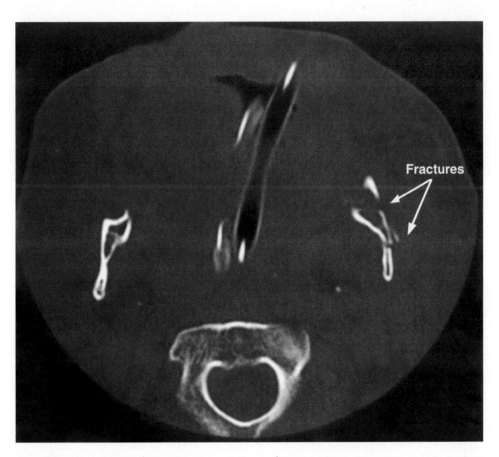

FIGURE 5-19   Mandible fracture seen on CT scan. *(Courtesy Summa Health System, Akron, Ohio.)*

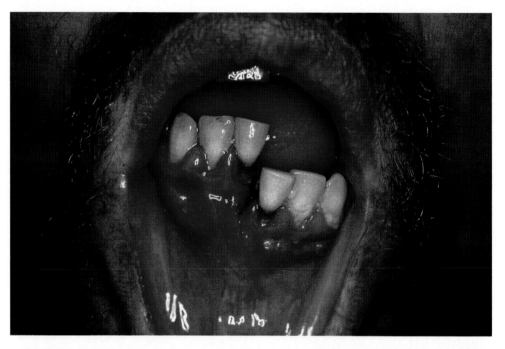

FIGURE 5-20   Steps in teeth. *(Courtesy Dr. David Effron, MetroHealth Medical Center, Cleveland, Ohio.)*

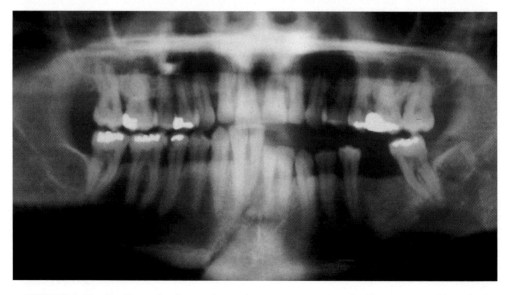

FIGURE 5-21   Radiograph of steps in teeth. *(Courtesy Dr. David Effron, MetroHealth Medical Center, Cleveland, Ohio.)*

a possible fracture. The patient should be asked whether his or her teeth seem to be coming together normally, because very commonly jaw fractures result in a disturbance of occlusion. The patient is then asked to open his or her mouth maximally and to move it from side to side maximally. The inability to open at least 35 mm or move side to side 6 mm leads to the suspicion of trismus caused by mandibular fracture or damage to the temporomandibular joint. As stated earlier, numbness of the lower lip is highly suspicious of a fracture and should be evaluated.

Dentition

All teeth must first be counted, and any missing teeth or parts of teeth must be documented and accounted for. If teeth cannot be found, intra-oral lacerations must be probed for their presence. If whole teeth or tooth fragments are still unaccounted for, chest and abdominal radiographs must be taken to rule out aspiration or ingestion.

Once all teeth are documented as being present or absent, each remaining tooth is tested for mobility. A singly mobile tooth may be the result of periodontal disease or root fracture or from lying in the line of a vertical fracture of the maxilla or mandible. Teeth that are mobile in groups are commonly associated with a segmental fracture of the maxilla, mandible, or alveolar bone of either. All such mobilities must be charted.

DIAGNOSING FACIAL TRAUMA

The following chart provides the examiner a quick reference guide for diagnosing oral and facial trauma based on clinical signs and symptomatology (Table 5-2).

RADIOLOGIC EVALUATION

Only after a complete clinical examination of the oral and facial trauma victim should diagnostic radiologic evaluation be considered. The reason is twofold: (1) an astute clinician will be able to detect most injuries clinically; and (2) a thorough examination will direct which specific radiologic surveys should be ordered.[2]

SUMMARY

Domestic violence injuries are frequently seen in the facial region. Because of this, appropriate assessment techniques are essential for identifying, documenting, and treating oral and facial trauma. This includes examination of the facial structures and soft tissue, pertinent cranial nerves, and the intra-oral cavity. Consultation with specialty services such as neurosurgery may be needed to rule out critical injury.

Table 5-2 Clinical Signs and Symptoms of Midfacial Fractures									
FRACTURE	ALVEOLAR	LE FORT I	LE FORT II	LE FORT III	ZYGOMATICO-MAXILLARY COMPLEX	ZYGOMATIC ARCH	ISOLATED NASAL	NASO-ORBITAL–ETHMOID	ORBITAL BLOWOUT
Airway obstruction	–	±	±	±	–	–	+	±	–
Asymmetry, facial	–	–	–	–	±	+	+	±	–
Cerebrospinal fluid leak	–	–	±	±	–	–	±	+	–
Crepitus	–	+	+	+	+	+	+	+	–
Decreased extraocular muscle function	–	–	±	±	±			±	±
Diplopia	–	–	±	±	±	–	–	±	±
Ecchymosis, buccal vestibule	+	+	+	–	+	–	–	–	–
Ecchymosis, periorbital	–	–	+	+	+	–	+	+	±
Ecchymosis, subconjunctival	–	–	+	+	+	–	±	+	±
Enophthalmos	–	–	±	±	±	–	–	–	±
Epistaxis, bilateral	–	+	+	+	–	–	+	+	–

Clinical finding	1	2	3	4	5	6	7	8	9
Epistaxis, unilateral	+	−	+	−	+|	−	−	−	−
Infraorbital rim defect	−	+	−	−	+|	−	+	−	−
Lateral orbital rim defect	−	−	−	−	+|	+	−	−	−
Lengthening of face	−	−	−	−	−	+	+	+|	−
Limitation of opening, trismus	−	−	−	+	+|	+|	+|	−	−
Malocclusion	−	−	−	−	−	+	+	+	+
Medial canthal deformity	−	+	−	−	−	+|	+|	−	−
Mobility of teeth	−	−	−	−	−	−	−	−	+
Nasal septal deformity	−	+|	+|	−	−	+|	+|	+|	−
Paresthesia, anterior cheek	+	−	−	−	+	+	+	+|	−
Pupil height, unequal	+|	−	−	−	+|	+|	+|	−	−

+, Consistent clinical finding; ±, possible finding; −, no clinical finding.

From Gerlock A.J. Jr, Sinn D.P., *Clinical and radiographic interpretation of facial fractures*, Boston, 1981, Little, Brown.

REFERENCES

1. Berrios DC, Grady D: Domestic violence: risk factors and outcomes, *West J Med* 155(2):133-135, 1991.
2. Fonseca R, Walker R: *Oral and maxillofacial trauma,* ed 2, Philadelphia, 1997, Saunders.
3. Gerlock AJ Jr, Sinn DP: *Clinical and radiographic interpretation of facial fractures,* Boston, 1981, Little, Brown.

SUGGESTED READING

Busuito MJ, Smith DJ, Robson MC: Mandibular fractures in an urban trauma center, *J Trauma* 26(9):826-829, 1986.

Fenton SJ, Bouquot JE, Unkel JH: Orofacial considerations for pediatric, adult and elderly victims of abuse, *Oral-Facial Emerg* 18(3):601-617, 2000.

Greene D and others: Epidemiology of facial injuries in blunt assault: determinants of incidence and outcome in 802 patients, *Arch Otolaryngol Head Neck Surg* 123(9):923-928, 1997.

Hartzell KN, Botek AA, Goldberg SH: Orbital fractures in women due to sexual assault and domestic violence, *Opthalmology* 103(6):954-957, 1996.

Kleinsasser NH and others: External trauma to the larynx: classification, diagnosis and therapy, *Eur Arch Otorhinolaryngol* 257:439-444, 2000.

Perciaccante VJ, Ochs HA, Dodson TB: Head, neck and facial injuries as markers of domestic violence in women, *J Oral Maxillofac Surg* 57:760-762, 1999.

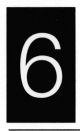

6 BLUNT THORACIC TRAUMA

Alan Markowitz • S. Scott Polsky • Jenifer Markowitz

In cases of domestic violence, injuries to the chest wall and its contents are not uncommon, especially because trauma may be targeted toward the breasts and other areas that are not visible when a person is fully clothed. Yeo[1] noted that only 45% of patients with thoracic trauma had injuries to the chest wall. Gunshot and other penetrating wounds require obvious referral; blunt trauma, however, is harder to assess and treat. This chapter examines the consequences of blunt chest trauma: rib injuries, lung contusions, associated hemopneumothorax, injuries to the heart and great vessels, and ruptured diaphragm.

Initial assessment should consider the victim's individual medical profile. An elderly victim of domestic abuse afflicted with rheumatoid arthritis on steroids may present a completely different picture than an otherwise healthy 28-year-old woman. Most importantly, common things *are* common: fractured ribs and pneumothorax occur far more frequently than injuries to the heart, lungs, esophagus, and diaphragm.

Abnormal breathing may result from serious chest wall injuries such as flail chest (Figure 6-1), pulmonary contusion (Figure 6-2), hemothorax (Figure 6-3), pneumothorax (Figure 6-4), tension pneumothorax (Figure 6-5), or ruptured diaphragm (Figure 6-6). Circulatory compromise may result from a hemothorax, tension pneumothorax, cardiac tamponade, or other cardiac injury. All these injuries may be found or suspected on a chest x-ray film.

CRITICAL CHEST INJURIES

The most critical injuries from blunt chest trauma include tension pneumothorax, rupture of the tracheobronchial tree, massive hemothorax, ruptured aorta or other great vessel, cardiac tamponade, and ruptured diaphragm. These injuries are usually the result of motor vehicle collisions and are rarely inflicted by interpersonal trauma unless the physical assault is exceedingly violent, as with a blunt object such as a baseball bat. The mechanism of trauma provides a key to the resultant injury and can direct the clinician beyond just a superficial ecchymosis on the chest wall. In summary, the mechanism of injury and the patient's medical history should guide the clinician in the determination of the extent of the workup.

Text continued on page 114

107

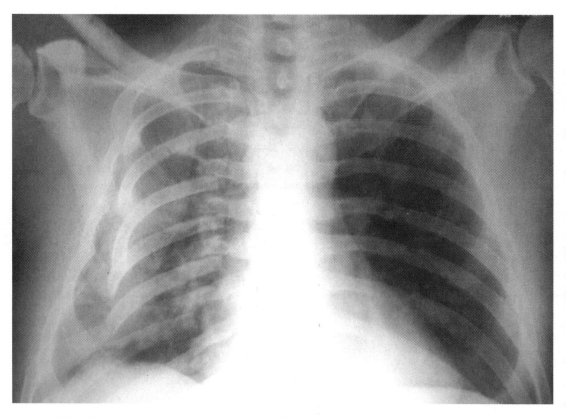

FIGURE 6-1   Multiple rib fractures with flail chest. *(Courtesy Dr. David Effron, MetroHealth Medical Center, Cleveland, Ohio.)*

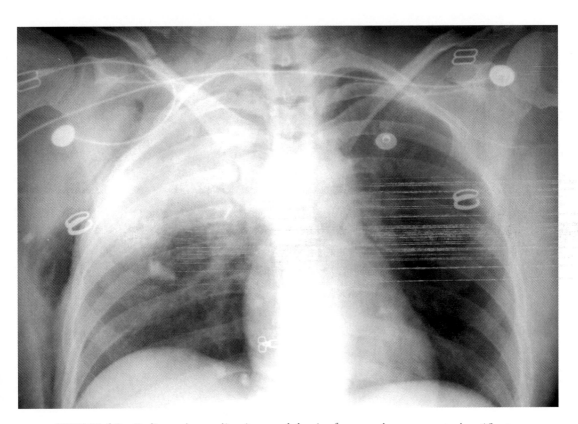

FIGURE 6-2   Radiograph revealing increased density from a pulmonary contusion. *(Courtesy Dr. David Effron, MetroHealth Medical Center, Cleveland, Ohio.)*

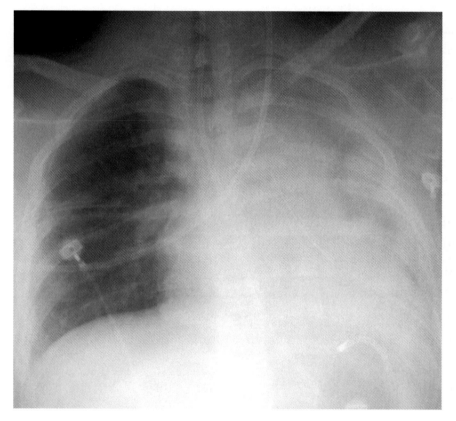

FIGURE 6-3 Radiograph revealing a hemothorax and rib fractures. *(Courtesy Dr. David Effron, MetroHealth Medical Center, Cleveland, Ohio.)*

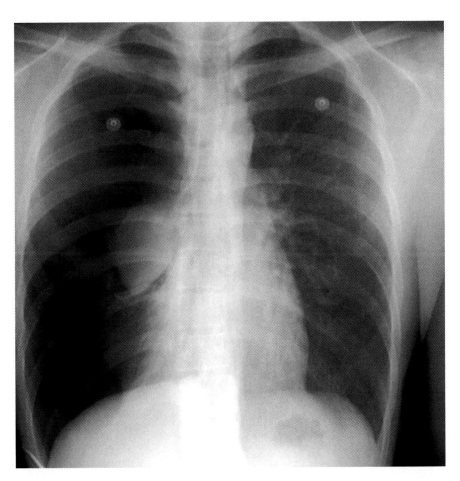

FIGURE 6-4   Radiograph of pneumothorax. *(Courtesy Dr. David Effron, MetroHealth Medical Center, Cleveland, Ohio.)*

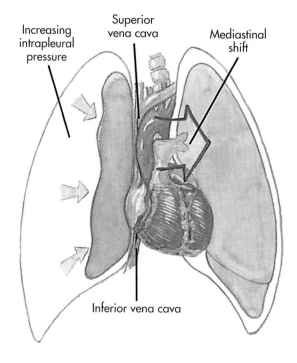

FIGURE 6-5   Diagram of tension pneumothorax. *(Sanders MJ, McKenna K:* Mosby's paramedic textbook, *ed 2, St. Louis, 2000, Mosby.)*

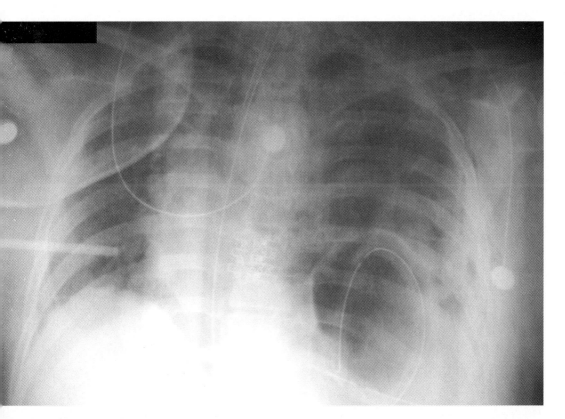

FIGURE 6-6   Radiograph showing the nasogastric tube in the chest cavity placed because of a ruptured diaphragm. *(Courtesy Dr. David Effron, MetroHealth Medical Center, Cleveland, Ohio.)*

Tracheobronchial Tree Injury

The patient will present with a tension pneumothorax, subcutaneous air, and hemoptysis; if a major airway is disrupted, the patient may die before reaching the hospital. Mediastinal air is visible on chest x-ray film, and there is frequently a persistent air leak after chest tube placement. Air can also escape into the mediastinum and be visible on x-ray film. The clinician may also hear "Hamman's crunch" on auscultation as the contracting heart "crunches" the mediastinal air wedged in between the pericardium and the lungs.

Pneumothorax

Severity of pneumothorax depends upon the amount of lung collapsed, unilateral or bilateral collapse, whether any "tension" exists, and if the tension is causing mediastinal displacement resulting in hemodynamic compromise (see Figure 6-7). Transgression of the visceral pleura allows positive-pressure air to enter the negative-pressure thorax; chest tube

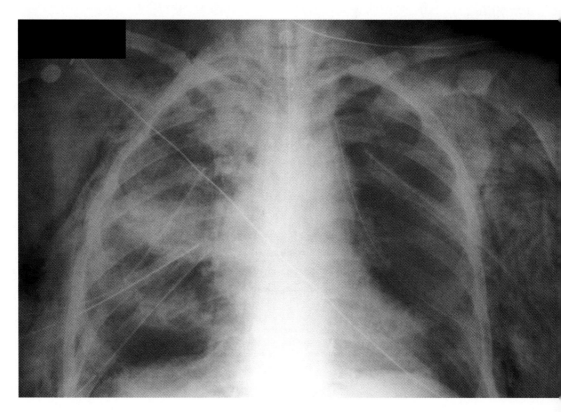

FIGURE 6-7   Mediastinal air and subcutaneous emphysema on chest radiograph. *(Courtesy Dr. David Effron, MetroHealth Medical Center, Cleveland, Ohio.)*

insertion will usually cure the problem as long as the production of air does not exceed the tube's ability to evacuate it. If the lung remains collapsed or the mediastinum remains shifted, the problem is more complicated and a thoracic surgical consult should be obtained. The vast majority of pneumothoraces can be treated by the initial chest tube placement (Figure 6-8).

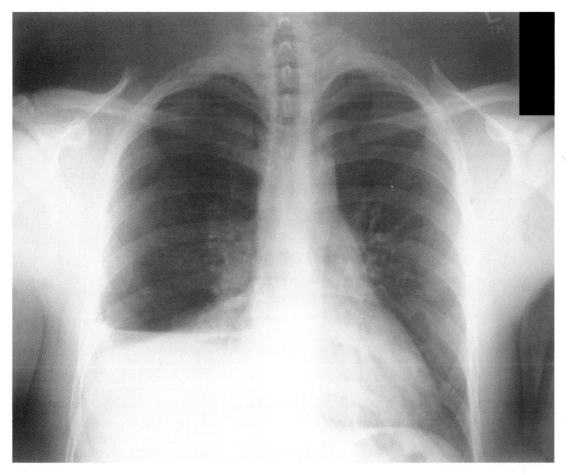

FIGURE 6-8 Hemopneumothorax. *(Courtesy Dr. David Effron, MetroHealth Medical Center, Cleveland, Ohio.)*

Rupture of a Great Vessel and Hemothorax

Rupture of a great vessel, primarily the aorta, will present with both shock and respiratory compromise. There is no external bleeding unless there are associated injuries, but chest x-ray will demonstrate a mediastinal hematoma (widening) or extensive hemothorax (Figure 6-9). Because this is an arterial hematoma, observation of tracheal or esophageal deviation would mandate immediate computed tomography (CT) scan. Not infrequently, patients with ruptured aortas wall off the leak, are hemodynamically uncompromised, and clinically appear stable, belying what lies underneath (see Figure 6-9).

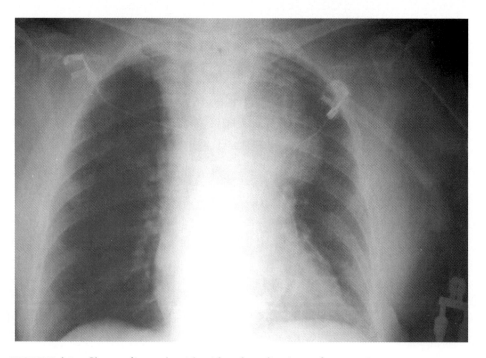

FIGURE 6-9   Chest radiograph with widened mediastinum from aortic aneurysm. *(Courtesy Dr. David Effron, MetroHealth Medical Center, Cleveland, Ohio.)*

Cardiac Injury and Tamponade

Penetrating injuries more commonly cause cardiac tamponade than blunt trauma. The diagnosis is suggested by Beck's triad: elevated venous pressure, decreased blood pressure, and diminished heart tones. Pulsus paradoxus, in which the systolic blood pressure drops by more than 10 mm Hg during inspiration (the opposite of normal), supports the diagnosis. Blunt trauma to the chest more commonly causes myocardial contusion, and actual rupture of a cardiac chamber or valve disruption are rare. These may all present with a dysrhythmia or cardiac failure and shock (Figure 6-10). Lindstaedt and others,[2] in a study of 118 patients with blunt thoracic trauma, found that 57% required admission to the surgical intensive care

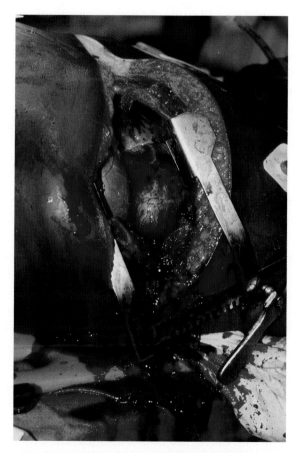

FIGURE 6-10 Tamponade. *(Courtesy Dr. David Effron, MetroHealth Medical Center, Cleveland, Ohio.)*

unit (ICU) as a result of their noncardiac injuries. Fourteen patients had myocardial contusions, 13 of which had been admitted to the ICU. None of these patients had acute cardiac complications in the hospital, and only 1 had new pathology on follow-up.[2]

EXAMINATION AND RADIOGRAPHS

Blunt chest trauma most frequently presents with local pain at the site of the injury and respiratory compromise. Every patient with stable vital signs should have a posterior-anterior (PA) and lateral chest x-ray examination to rule out trauma to the underlying lung. If the patient is unstable, an anterior-posterior (AP) portable chest x-ray will suffice. Separate rib detail films are necessary to assess rib fracture and displacement, an especially important consideration in the elderly with osteoporosis. If respiratory compromise is disproportionate to the extent of the injury, arterial blood gases (ABGs) should be obtained and a chest CT scan should be performed because significant trauma to the underlying lung may have been missed. Observing the patient's ventilatory efforts and chest wall motion are important features of the physical examination to alert the clinician to underlying problems. Diminished breath sounds and rales in the region of blunt trauma are often found, signifying pulmonary contusion. This reflects either blunt trauma to the lung parenchyma itself or intraparenchymal hemorrhage. Both would alert the clinician to admit the patient for observation and expectant treatment. Otherwise healthy patients should be able to heal most of this with relatively little support. Elderly patients and those with underlying pulmonary disease or immunocompromise may have much more difficulty and should be admitted for observation to ensure that infectious complications do not supervene.

RIB AND PULMONARY INJURIES AND FLAIL CHEST

Bruised or fractured ribs are the most common blunt traumatic injury to the chest. The consequences are dictated by the patient's age; the pediatric rib cage is largely cartilaginous, and children may have significant bruising without actual fractures. Adults, with a firm bony matrix, will fracture more easily, and it is most critical to detect any bony displacement of the rib fracture. Inward displacement of a rib shard could result in severe hemorrhage both into the lung substance itself and into the pleural space, which may not stop until the rib fragment is removed. Flail chest occurs when two or more adjacent ribs are each fractured in two or more places causing paradoxical movement of a segment of the chest during breathing. During inspiration, when the chest wall normally expands, the segment retracts, and during expiration it moves outward (Figures 6-11 and 6-12). This decreases air movement, and in the presence of a lung contusion may produce severe respiratory compromise. Elderly patients with osteoporosis and calcified costal cartilages present a somewhat brittle rib cage to blunt trauma and may have extensive fractures disproportionate to the actual trauma itself. The elderly are more prone to inward displacement of a fractured rib. Complete assessment of these patients includes CT scanning, especially in a patient with a respiratory problem disproportionate to the injury.

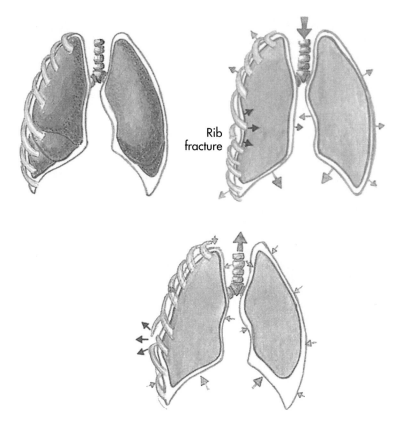

Rib
fracture

FIGURE 6-11 Diagram of a flail chest. *(Sanders MJ, McKenna K:* Mosby's paramedic textbook, *ed 2, St. Louis, 2000, Mosby.)*

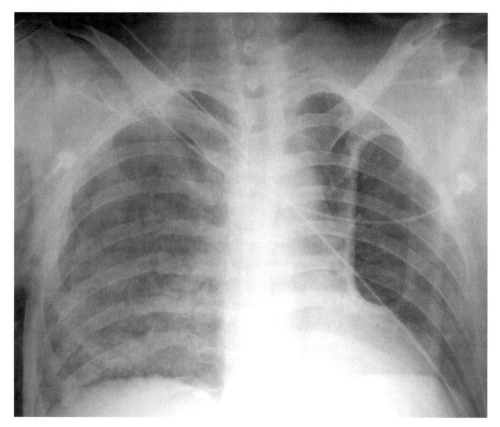

FIGURE 6-12   Radiograph of flail chest. *(Courtesy Dr. David Effron, MetroHealth Medical Center, Cleveland, Ohio.)*

In chest trauma analysis, the clinician must always be aware of the patient's medical history. Does this patient have disease that may predispose him or her to developing complications from what was thought to be minor blunt chest wall trauma? The most important observation is ease of ventilation. If the patient breathes easily without pain and with normal frequency, he or she is not likely to encounter problems later if no anatomic injuries are identified. However, the clinician's suspicions should be aroused if there are medical problems in the background: uncontrolled glucose in a diabetic patient, immunosuppressive medications, chronic steroid ingestion, etc. Admission to a hospital for 24-hour observation with a second chest x-ray film obtained 12 hours after the first encounter will likely detect complications that would have eluded attention had the patient been discharged. A good history, with close attention to the mechanism of injury, and careful physical examination of the patient's respiratory status and mechanics of inhalation will catch most underlying problems. Can the patient breathe deeply, or is she limited by pain? Has she coughed up any blood? Does he feel like he can ventilate himself adequately, or is he constantly searching for air? Has she had any lung problems in the past? If any of these are concerns, PA and lateral chest x-ray films and ABGs will alert the clinician that there is further cause for concern. If the chest x-ray film is equivocal in the face of a persistently symptomatic patient, chest CT will provide additional information that can be easily missed on chest x-ray.

The most frequently missed injuries resulting from domestic violence are traumatic pneumo-hemothorax and internal displacement of fractured ribs. Occult bleeding resulting from displaced rib fractures can create catastrophic complications, even cardiac arrest. The presence of a small hemothorax, although not requiring a chest tube, should be the grounds for admission and observation with serial chest x-rays to rule out further accumulation. If a pneumothorax is 20% or less, a standard chest tube is not required and a smaller 16- to 20-French cannula can be placed and attached to a one-way Heimlich valve, usually with resolution of the pneumothorax. If there is significant collection of air and blood, a standard chest tube should be placed and hooked to suction; serial chest x-ray films should be obtained over the next 12 hours to determine the stability of the injury.

REFERENCES

1. Yeo TP: Long-term sequelae following blunt thoracic trauma, *Orthoped Nurs* 20(5):35-47, 2001.
2. Lindstaedt M and others: Acute and long-term clinical significance of myocardial contusion following blunt thoracic trauma: results of a prospective study, *J Trauma* 52(3):479-485, 2002.

SUGGESTED READING

Bokhari F and others: Prospective evaluation of the sensitivity of physical examination in chest trauma, *J Trauma* 53(6):1135-1138, 2002.
Gavelli G and others: Traumatic injuries: image of thoracic injuries, *Eur Radiol* 12(6):1273-1294, 2002.

7 BLUNT ABDOMINAL TRAUMA

S. Scott Polsky

ASSESSMENT

Abdominal trauma from domestic violence frequently results from blunt force, such as blows or stomping incidents. Particularly common are injuries to the liver, spleen, and kidneys.[1] All abdominal pain following blunt trauma should be taken seriously, regardless of whether there are external indicators of the blunt force, such as contusions or patterned injury from weapons. Imaging is of particular importance in abdominal blunt trauma. Poletti and others, in their review of the literature, report that clinical findings are equivocal or misleading in 20% to 50% of patients presenting with blunt polytrauma.[2]

Patients who exhibit signs of hypotension or signs of peritoneal irritation such as involuntary guarding and rebound should be seen at a hospital capable of handling trauma. Any significant abdominal tenderness requires at least serial examinations over several hours and often requires further specific testing. The *Kehr sign* is referred pain to the left shoulder from irritation of the diaphragm. It may indicate a splenic injury and requires a surgical consult. Physical examination may also reveal abdominal distention from ileus or pneumoperitoneum. Blood alone, however, will not result in visible enlargement of abdominal girth. Ecchymosis may be apparent from subcutaneous bleeding in any part of the body. Particular attention must be paid to ecchymosis at the umbilicus *(Cullen sign)* (Figure 7-1) or at the flanks *(Turner sign),* which indicates retroperitoneal bleeding. Tenderness over the lower thorax may indicate rib fractures, which can have associated injuries to the liver, spleen, and kidneys. Renal injury is more likely to be seen in blunt trauma than penetrating trauma, although blunt trauma does not inflict the magnitude of injury brought about by penetrating trauma.[3] Less common, pancreatic injury may also be present, although rarely as an isolated event.[4] Pelvic fractures should be suspected if there is tenderness on palpation, pain with pelvic compression, or instability of the pelvis on examination (Figure 7-2).

Simple abdominal radiographs have limited value in assessing blunt abdominal trauma. Free air may be visible under the diaphragm when a hollow viscus has ruptured (Figure 7-3). Ileus is often present but is nonspecific and helps little in patient management. Ultrasound (US) is used in many institutions directly in the emergency department to assess for the presence of

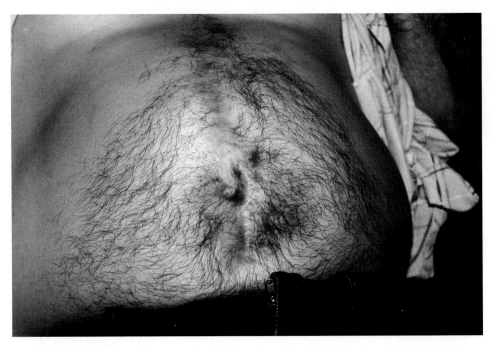

FIGURE 7-1   Cullen sign. *(Courtesy Dr. David Effron, MetroHealth Medical Center, Cleveland, Ohio.)*

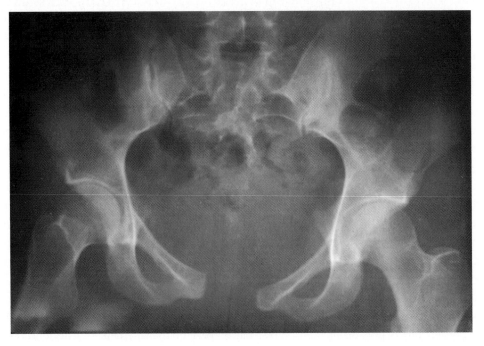

FIGURE 7-2   Pelvic fracture. *(Courtesy Trauma Services, Summa Health System, Akron, Ohio.)*

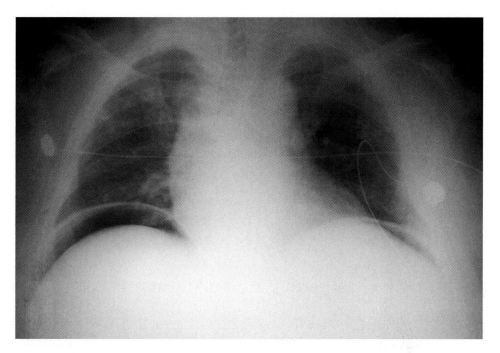

FIGURE 7-3   Radiograph of free air in the chest cavity. *(Courtesy Dr. David Effron, MetroHealth Medical Center, Cleveland, Ohio.)*

blood in the peritoneum (Figure 7-4) and cardiac tamponade. It is, in fact, the method of choice for initial screening for free abdominal fluid and parenchymal injuries.[2] For many years peritoneal lavage was considered the gold standard for assessing the need for immediate surgery for intraperitoneal injuries. Computerized tomography (CT) scanning offers the advantages of visualizing retroperitoneal injuries, providing organ-specific diagnosis, and identifying significant injuries that may not require immediate surgery (Figures 7-5 and 7-6). There is some evidence that the routine use of FAST (focused assessment with sonography for trauma) for blunt abdominal injury is a more efficient and less expensive method for diagnosis than CT or diagnostic peritoneal lavage and appears to have comparable accuracy.[5] However, CT requires less dependence on operator skill and has greater reproducibility.[2]

TREATMENT

The key element in treating blunt abdominal trauma is determining the need for emergent surgical intervention. The American College of Surgeons recommends that patients with potentially severe injuries be transferred to trauma centers (Box 7-1). If the patient is being transferred from another facility (hospital, physician's office, or minor care center), he or she must be stabilized before transport. If the patient's condition is potentially unstable, the physician must document that the benefits of transfer outweigh the risks. The patient must be

Text continued on page 130

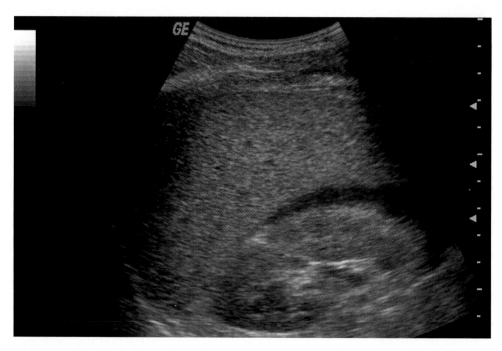

FIGURE 7-4 Ultrasound of free fluid in the abdomen. *(Courtesy Dr. David Effron, MetroHealth Medical Center, Cleveland, Ohio.)*

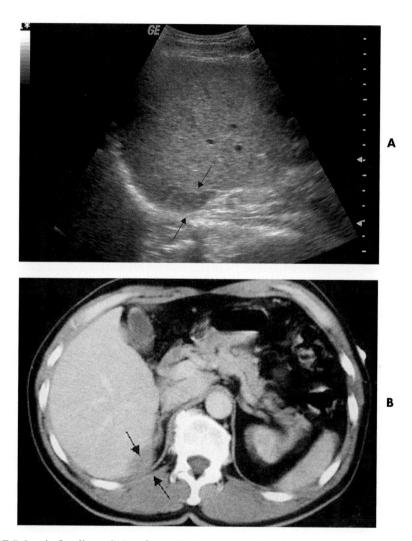

FIGURE 7-5   **A,** Small anechoic subcapsular hematoma of the liver *(arrows).* **B,** CT image of same patient with subcapsular hematoma *(arrows). (Courtesy Dr. Robert Jones, MetroHealth Medical Center, Cleveland, Ohio.)*

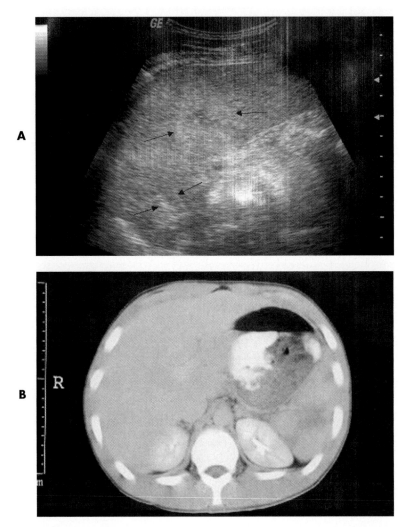

FIGURE 7-6   **A,** Splenic laceration/hematoma *(arrows).* **B,** CT image of same patient with splenic laceration/hematoma *(arrows). (Courtesy Dr. Robert Jones, MetroHealth Medical Center, Cleveland, Ohio.)*

Box 7-1	*Interhospital Transfer Criteria* When the Patient's Needs Exceed Available Resources

CLINICAL CIRCUMSTANCES

Central Nervous System
- Head injury
  - Penetrating injury or depressed skull fracture
  - Open injury with or without CSF leak
  - GCS score 14 or GCS deterioration
  - Lateralizing signs
  - Spinal cord injury or major vertebral injury

Chest
- Widened mediastinum or signs suggesting great vessel injury
- Major chest wall injury or pulmonary contusion
- Cardiac injury
- Patients who may require prolonged ventilation

Pelvis/Abdomen
- Unstable pelvic-ring disruption
- Pelvic-ring disruption with shock and evidence of continuing hemorrhage
- Open pelvic injury

Extremity
- Severe open fractures
- Traumatic amputation with potential for replantation
- Complex articular fractures
- Major crush injury
- Ischemia

Multisystem Injury
- Head injury with face, chest, abdominal, or pelvic injury
- Injury to more than two body regions
- Major burns or burns with associated injuries
- Multiple proximal long-bone fractures

Comorbid Factors
- Age >55 years
- Children
- Cardiac or respiratory disease
- Insulin-dependent diabetes
- Morbid obesity
- Pregnancy
- Immunosuppression

Secondary Deterioration (Late Sequelae)
- Mechanical ventilation required
- Sepsis
- Single or multiple organ system failure (deterioration in central nervous, cardiac, pulmonary, hepatic, renal, or coagulation system)
- Major tissue necrosis

Modified from ACS Committee on Trauma: *Resources for optimal care of the injured patient,* 1997, The Committee.[5]
CSF, Cerebrospinal fluid; *GCS,* Glasgow Coma Scale.

transferred utilizing the highest level of emergency medical services (EMS) transport available, and all transfers must comply with the Emergency Medical Treatment and Labor Act (EMTALA) requirements.

SUMMARY AND CONCLUSIONS

Domestic violence events such as stomping or striking can result in significant intraabdominal injury and should be conservatively evaluated. Diagnostic imaging is essential, because physical examination alone may not adequately reveal the full extent of the injury. Clinicians should remember, however, that acute injury would not be the only reason patients experiencing domestic violence will present with abdominal pain. In fact, abdominal pain and functional abdominal disorders are common in this population and should be taken no less seriously than acute injury.[6-8]

REFERENCES

1. Jurkovich GJ, Carrico CJ: Pancreatic trauma, *Surg Clin North Am* 70:575-593, 1990.
2. Poletti PA and others: Traumatic injuries: role of imaging in the management of the polytrauma victim, *Eur Radiol* 12(5):969-978, 2002.
3. Dreitlein DA, Suner S, Basler J: Genitourinary trauma, *Emerg Med Clin North Am* 19(3):569-590, 2001.
4. Higashitani K and others: Complete transection of the pancreas due to a single stamping injury: a case report, *Int J Legal Med* 115(2):72-75, 2001.
5. Boulanger BR and others: Prospective evidence of the superiority of a sonography-based algorithm in the assessment of blunt abdominal injury, *J Trauma* 47(4):632-637.
6. Drossman DA and others: Sexual and physical abuse in women with functional or organic gastrointestinal disorders, *Ann Intern Med* 113(11):828-833, 1990.
7. Campbell J and others: Intimate partner violence and physical health consequences, *Arch Intern Med* 162:1157-1163, 2002.
8. Markowitz JR: *Care of the abused patient within a forensic nursing framework,* Paper presented at the Women and Medicine Conference: Northeast Ohio Universities College of Medicine, Rootstown, Ohio, April 2002.
9. ACS Committee on Trauma: *Resources for optimal care of the injured patient,* 1997, The Committee

TRAUMA IN PREGNANCY

Justin Lavin, Jr.

Domestic violence has been reported to occur in 1% to 20% of pregnancies.[1,2] In most studies the prevalence clusters in the 4%-to-8% range.[1-3] However, rates appear to be higher among younger patients, indigent women, those who smoke or use illicit drugs, gravidas who delay seeking prenatal care, and women with unintended pregnancies.[1,3-7] More than 20% of victims have reported an increase in assaults during pregnancy.[3,8] Approximately 25% of abused pregnant women report having been struck in the abdomen.[3,8] The best predicator of domestic violence in pregnancy is a history of similar assault before pregnancy.[5] Of women who suffer such abuse during pregnancy, 88% have a history of domestic violence preceding the pregnancy.[5,9] As other causes of maternal mortality have declined, violence has become a proportionally more important cause of maternal death.[10,11] In a recent study from North Carolina, 51.2% of women who were murdered during pregnancy were assaulted by their spouse or partner and 40% of suicide fatalities were known or suspected to be abused.[11] Others have reported increased maternal complications including chorioamnionitis, urinary tract infection, and cesarean delivery.[3,12]

The overall effect of domestic violence on fetal and neonatal health is more difficult to define. Some authors have reported increased preterm labor, decreased birth weights, and increased prevalence of neonatal intensive care unit (NICU) admissions.[3,13-15] However, when correcting for other risk factors such as socioeconomic status, age, smoking, and drug abuse, other investigators have not observed all or some of these effects.[3,16-18] Although it is difficult to precisely quantify the varied contribution of all of the factors just mentioned, women who experience domestic violence clearly constitute a group at high risk for adverse neonatal outcomes.[3,13,14,16-18] In addition, as with any type of trauma, domestic violence has been associated with direct fetal injury, abruption, premature labor, and stillbirth.[3,12,19,20] With life-threatening maternal trauma, fetal loss rates have approached 40% to 50%, whereas with non–life-threatening maternal injury, fetal loss rates have been reported to range from 1% to 5%.[21,22] However, because non–life-threatening injury is much more common, the majority of trauma-related fetal losses occur in such cases.[21-25]

ANATOMY, PHYSIOLOGY, AND INJURY PATTERNS OF PREGNANCY

The anatomic and physiologic changes of pregnancy may affect the pattern and presentation of injuries sustained by the pregnant victim of domestic violence. Maternal cardiac output increases and peaks at about 40% above baseline near the end of the second trimester.[26] Maternal heart rate increases by 15%, with rates of 80 to 95 beats per minute (bpm) falling within the normal range.[26] Blood pressure decreases by 5 to 15 mm Hg in the second trimester and returns to normal in the third trimester. If the mother lies flat on her back, compression of the maternal vena cava and aorta by the weight of the gravid uterus may result in supine hypotension.[26] Maternal blood volume is increased by approximately 1000 ml. Because plasma volume increases to a greater extent than red cell mass, hemoglobin may decrease slightly, with values as low as 10 g/dl being normal.[26,27] Because of her expanded blood volume, a gravid woman may be able to tolerate up to a 1500-ml blood loss before developing hypotension. However, she may maintain her own perfusion by shunting blood away from her uterus, which may in turn lead to fetal hypoxia.[26] These changes combine to cause the signs and symptoms commonly associated with shock to be difficult to interpret. In addition, they render appropriate judgments regarding fluid and blood replacement more complex[26,27] (Table 8-1).

Gastric motility is decreased and gastric emptying time increased in pregnant patients. Therefore if an injured pregnant woman becomes unconscious, she may be at increased risk for aspiration.[26,27] By its very nature, pregnancy induces marked changes in the genitourinary tract. In the first trimester, the uterus is largely confined to the pelvis and usually shielded from direct injury.[26] At the beginning of the second trimester, the uterus rises into the abdomen. Thereafter it may be ruptured by seemingly mild or innocuous blunt trauma or penetrated as a result of stabbing or gunshot wounds[26,27] (Figure 8-1). Because uterine blood flow is increased to 600 ml/min, laceration or rupture may result in rapid exsanguinations.[27] Uterine trauma may also result in direct fetal injury, premature labor, and/or abruption[25-28] (Figure 8-2). The enlarging uterus displaces the bowel into the upper abdomen. Therefore bowel injuries are less likely to occur with penetrating injuries to the lower abdomen, but penetration of the upper abdomen may result in multiple and severe bowel injuries.[25-27] The bladder is passively pulled

Table 8-1	*Physiologic Changes of Pregnancy*	
	SECOND TRIMESTER	THIRD TRIMESTER
Cardiac output	Increases 40%	
Heart rate	Increases 15%	
Blood pressure	Decreases 5-15 mm Hg	Normal
Blood volume		Increases 1000 ml
Hemoglobin		May decrease to 10 g/dl
Hypotension		May require 1500-ml blood loss

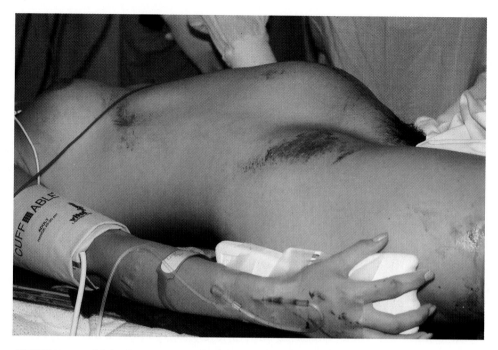

FIGURE 8-1   Multiple pelvic and chest abrasions. *(Courtesy Dr. David Effron, MetroHealth Medical Center, Cleveland, Ohio.)*

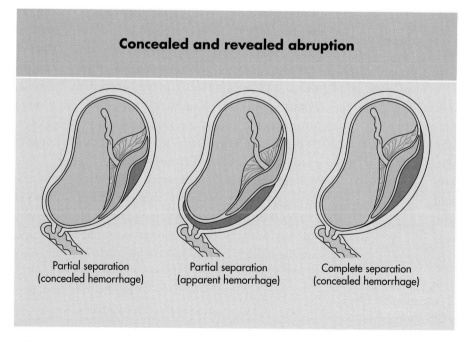

FIGURE 8-2   Concealed and revealed abruption. *(From Greer I, Cameron I, Kitchner H, Prentice A: Mosby's color atlas of obstetrics and gynecology, ed 1, St. Louis, 2001 Mosby.)*

upward by the expanding uterus and also becomes a more frequent site of injury.[26,27] The blood vessels supplying the pelvic organs expand dramatically. Therefore pelvic fractures causing vessel injury may result in dramatic concealed retroperitoneal bleeding.[25,26]

TREATMENT

Battered women constitute 22% to 35% of women seeking care in emergency departments.[29-31] A similar proportion of women presenting with injuries during pregnancy have been assaulted by a partner or spouse.[28,32] Minor maternal injuries may be treated expeditiously. However, the optimal management of a seriously injured pregnant victim of domestic violence is best accomplished by a multidisciplinary team involving emergency department physicians, obstetricians, trauma surgeons, emergency and obstetrical nurses, and associated personnel.[25,26]

Initial care should concentrate on assessing and maintaining an adequate airway, breathing, and circulation.[25-27] An airway should be secured and maintained.[25-27] If the patient is unconscious, this is best accomplished by rapid-sequence induction with cricoid pressure to avoid gastric aspiration.[27] Supplemental oxygen should be administered.[25-27] Hemoglobin oxygen saturation should be maintained at 90% or greater.[25] Whenever there is a question of severe injury or substantial blood loss, two large-bore intravenous (IV) lines should be placed.[25-27] At the time of insertion, blood should be obtained for complete blood count, platelet count, prothrombin time, partial thromboplastin time, fibrinogen, fibrin split products, electrolytes, liver function tests, blood urea nitrogen, creatinine, amylase, type and cross-match, and a Kleihauer-Betke test.[26] Crystalloid in the form of lactated Ringer's solution or normal saline should initially be used to replace blood loss in a 3:1 ratio.[25-27] If necessary, type-specific or type O-negative blood may be used, although transfusion of cross-matched Rh-negative compatible blood is preferable to complete blood replacement.[25-27] If possible, vasopressors should be avoided because they may reduce uterine blood flow.[25-27] However, they should not be withheld if urgently needed to resuscitate the mother.[25] The woman should be tilted to the left to minimize aortocaval compression and resultant hypotension.[25-27] If the mother must be kept supine for cardiopulmonary resuscitation (CPR) or assessment of spinal injury, the uterus should be manually displaced to the left.[25]

Once initial stabilization is complete, a diligent search to identify the extent of other injuries should be completed.[25-27] The pregnant abdomen is a frequent target of blows and stab and gunshot wounds. Therefore it should be carefully inspected for signs of blunt trauma, entrance and exit wounds, and internal injury. Blows may result in extensive organ injury and bleeding.[25-27] Abdominal lavage may be indicated if abdominal trauma results in signs suggestive of intraperitoneal bleeding, altered sensorium, unexplained shock, major thoracic injuries, or multiple major orthopedic injuries.[25,26] An open procedure is usually preferred after the first trimester to minimize the risk of injury.[25-27] Computed tomography (CT) scan may also be helpful.[25,27] This procedure results in approximately 3.5 rads exposure to the fetus.[25] Because 20 to 25 rads is required to cause significant risk of fetal injury, it and other necessary x-rays should not be withheld.[25-27] All x-rays should still be carefully planned to minimize exposure.[25,26] If stab wounds do not penetrate the peritoneum, they often may be treated conservatively.[25-27] Those stab wounds that may penetrate the peritoneum, and gunshot wounds require laparotomy.[25-27] X-ray films from multiple projections may help to localize the bullet.[25,26] A Foley catheter should be placed to assess urine output.[25-27] Substantially bloody urine or difficulty with insertion may indicate bladder injury and requires further evaluation.[25-27] Pelvic and extremity fractures should be stabilized.[25-27]

FETAL ASSESSMENT AND INJURIES

As soon as the mother has been stabilized, attention should turn to fetal evaluation.[25-28,32] This is true even if maternal injuries do not appear extensive. Although, generally, the probability of fetal death is correlated with the maternal Injury Severity Score, fetal injury is relatively common even with a maternal Injury Severity Score of zero.[32] Extreme uterine tenderness or vaginal bleeding may suggest abruption or uterine rupture.[25,26] Speculum examination should be performed to rule out unapparent bleeding or amniotic fluid leakage.[26] If the fetus has reached 22 to 24 weeks' gestation, making it potentially viable, electronic fetal heart rate monitoring should be instituted.[25-27] An abnormal fetal heart rate may indicate the need for cesarean in the fetal interest.[25-27] At more than 20 weeks' gestation, contraction monitoring should be carried out for a minimum of 4 to 6 hours.[25,28,33-35] Frequent contractions (more than 6 per hour) may suggest an increased risk of abruption[24,33] or premature labor. If such contractions are present, monitoring and observation should be continued for 24 to 72 hours because of the risk of delayed abruption.[25,34] The patient should also be assessed for menstrual-like cramping, low back pain, vaginal bleeding, or rupture of membranes.

An individual experienced in assessment of fetal and placental anatomy should perform an ultrasound.[25,27] During this procedure, the fetal skull, spine, ribs, and extremities should be searched for potential fracture. The fetal brain, chest, and abdomen should also be evaluated for signs of bleeding. The placenta should be assessed for retroplacental clot, tearing, unusual thickening, or elevation of the membranes on contralateral sides of the uterus that may suggest a concealed abruption (Figure 8-3). Kleihauer-Betke testing may also help detect concealed fetal-maternal bleeding.[25-27] If there is any question of fetal-to-maternal bleeding, Rh_o(D) immune globulin should be administered.[25-27] Because 90% of fetal-to-maternal hemorrhages caused by trauma result in the injection of less than 15 ml of fetal blood, one 300-μg vial of Rh_o(D) immune globulin will usually be sufficient.[24,36] In the rare instance in which a larger dose is required, it should be calculated based on the Kleihauer-Betke results.[25]

Very rarely, a woman may be battered too severely to survive her injuries.[10,11] In such cases, perimortem cesarean may be appropriate.[25,26] Prognosis for fetal survival is excellent if the cesarean delivery is less than 5 minutes after the mother's demise; good, if within 5 to 10 minutes; fair if within 10 to 15 minutes; and poor if longer than 15 minutes.[25,26,37]

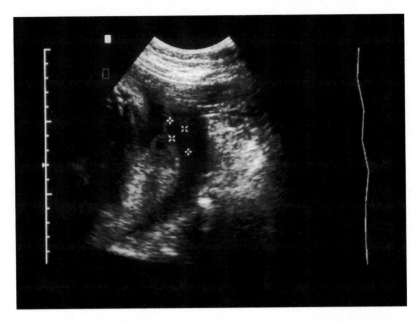

FIGURE 8-3   Placental abruption. *(Courtesy Dr. Justin Lavin, Akron General Medical Center and Summa Health Center, Akron, Ohio.)*

FOLLOW-UP

Once the mother's physical injuries have been treated and fetal well-being has been ensured, her emotional status and need for physical protection should be addressed.[28,32] Because many women are reluctant to admit abuse, formal screening is more productive.[1,38] It is important for the clinician to recognize that any pregnant woman may be a potential victim of abuse regardless or age, race, or marital or socioeconomic status.[1,32] Substance abuse, multiple emergency department visits, late or nonexistent prenatal care, unintended pregnancy, depression, or prior abuse should increase the clinician's suspicion.[1,3-11,32]

The pattern of physical injuries may also suggest interpersonal violence.[32] Injuries as a result of battery are frequently located around the head and neck.[32] Bruises of the breast, abdomen, and upper extremities may indicate domestic violence during pregnancy[3,8,32,39] as may injuries at multiple sites in varying stages of healing.[32] The trauma should be acknowledged.[1] The women's wishes should be respected, but her immediate safety should be evaluated.[1,28,32] Housing and shelter options should be addressed. Social service, advocacy groups, and shelter organizations may be helpful in these efforts.[1,28,32] In the rare instance in which no other alternative is available, short-term hospital admission may be appropriate.[1]

REFERENCES

1. American College of Obstetricians and Gynecologists: *Domestic violence,* Washington, DC, 1999, The College.
2. Gazmararian JA and others: Prevalence of violence against pregnant women, *JAMA* 275(24):1915-1920, 1996.
3. Berenson AB and others: Perinatal morbidity associated with violence experienced by pregnant women, *Am J Obstet Gynecol* 170(6):1760-1766; discussion 1766-1769, 1994.
4. Gazmararian JA and others: The relationship between pregnancy intendedness and physical violence in mothers of newborns: The PRAMS Working Group, *Obstet Gynecol* 85(6):1031-1038, 1995.
5. Glander SS and others: The prevalence of domestic violence among women seeking abortion, *Obstet Gynecol* 91(6):1002-1006, 1998.
6. McFarlane J and others: Assessing for abuse during pregnancy: severity and frequency of injuries and associated entry into prenatal care, *JAMA* 267(23):3176-3178, 1992.
7. Dietz PM and others: Delayed entry into prenatal care: effect of physical violence, *Obstet Gynecol* 90(2):221-224, 1997.
8. Berenson AB and others: Drug abuse and other risk factors for physical abuse in pregnancy among white non-Hispanic, black, and Hispanic women, *Am J Obstet Gynecol* 164(6 Pt 1):1491-1496; discussion 1496-1499, 1991.
9. Helton AS, McFarlane J, Anderson ET: Battered and pregnant: a prevalence study, *Am J Public Health* 77(10):1337-1339, 1987.
10. Dannenberg AL and others: Homicide and other injuries as causes of maternal death in New York City, 1987 through 1991, *Am J Obstet Gynecol* 172(5):1557-1564, 1995.
11. Parsons LH, Harper MA: Violent maternal deaths in North Carolina, *Obstet Gynecol* 94(6):990-993, 1999.
12. Cokkinides VE and others: Physical violence during pregnancy: maternal complications and birth outcomes, *Obstet Gynecol* 93(5 Pt 1):661-666, 1999.
13. Bullock LF, McFarlane J: The birth-weight/battering connection, *Am J Nurs* 89(9):1153-1155, 1989.
14. Schei B, Samuelsen SO, Bakketeig LS: Does spousal physical abuse affect the outcome of pregnancy? *Scand J Soc Med* 19(1):26-31, 1991.
15. Parker B, McFarlane J, Soeken K: Abuse during pregnancy: effects on maternal complications and birth weight in adult and teenage women, *Obstet Gynecol* 84(3):323-328, 1994.
16. Amaro H and others: Violence during pregnancy and substance use, *Am J Public Health* 80(5):575-579, 1990.
17. Grimstad H and others: Physical abuse and low birthweight: a case-control study, *Br J Obstet Gynaecol* 104(11):1281-1287, 1997.
18. O'Campo P and others: Verbal abuse and physical violence among a cohort of low-income pregnant women, *Women's Health Issues* 4(1):29-37, 1994.
19. Morey MA, Begleiter ML, Harris DJ: Profile of a battered fetus, *Lancet* 2(8258):1294-1295, 1981.
20. Sokal MM and others: Neonatal survival after traumatic fetal subdural hematoma, *J Reprod Med* 24(3):131-133, 1980.
21. Pearlman MD, Tintinalli JE: Evaluation and treatment of the gravida and fetus following trauma during pregnancy, *Obstet Gynecol Clin North Am* 18(2):371-381, 1991.
22. American College of Obstetricians and Gynecologists: *Obstetric aspects of trauma management,* Washington, DC, 1998, The College.
23. Fries MH, Hankins GD: Motor vehicle accident associated with minimal maternal trauma but subsequent fetal demise, *Ann Emerg Med* 18(3):301-304, 1989.
24. Pearlman MD, Tintinalli JE, Lorenz RP: Blunt trauma during pregnancy, *N Engl J Med* 323(23):1609-1613, 1990.
25. American College of Obstetricians and Gynecologists: *Vaginal birth after previous cesarean delivery,* Washington DC, 1998, The College.
26. Lavin JP Jr, Polsky SS: Abdominal trauma during pregnancy, *Clin Perinatol* 10(2):423-438, 1983.
27. Coleman MT, Trianfo VA, Rund DA: Nonobstetric emergencies in pregnancy: trauma and surgical conditions, *Am J Obstet Gynecol* 177(3):497-502, 1997.
28. Pak LL, Reece EA, Chan L: Is adverse pregnancy outcome predictable after blunt abdominal trauma? *Am J Obstet Gynecol* 179(5):1140-1144, 1998.
29. Goldberg WG, Tomlanovich MD: Domestic violence victims in the emergency department, *JAMA* 251(24):3259-3264, 1984.
30. McLeer SV and others: Education is not enough: a systems failure in protecting battered women, *Ann Emerg Med* 18(6):651-653, 1989.

31. American Medical Association: *Diagnostic and treatment guidelines on domestic violence,* Chicago, 1992, The Association.

32. Poole GV and others: Trauma in pregnancy: the role of interpersonal violence, *Am J Obstet Gynecol* 174(6):1873-1877; discussion 1877-1878, 1996.

33. Pearlman MD, Tintinalli JE, Lorenz RP: A prospective controlled study of outcome after trauma during pregnancy, *Am J Obstet Gynecol* 162(6):1502-1507; discussion 1507-1510, 1990.

34. Dahmus MA, Sibai BM: Blunt abdominal trauma: are there any predictive factors for abruptio placentae or maternal-fetal distress? *Am J Obstet Gynecol* 169(4):1054-1059, 1993.

35. American Academy of Pediatrics and American College of Obstetricians and Gynecologists: *Guidelines for perinatal care,* ed 4, Elk Grove Village, Ill, 1997, The Academy.

36. Goodwin TM, Breen MT: Pregnancy outcome and fetomaternal hemorrhage after noncatastrophic trauma, *Am J Obstet Gynecol* 162(3):665-671, 1990.

37. Weber CE: Postmortem cesarean section: review of the literature and case reports, *Am J Obstet Gynecol* 110(2):158-165, 1971.

38. Parsons LH and others: Methods of and attitudes toward screening obstetrics and gynecology patients for domestic violence, *Am J Obstet Gynecol* 173(2):381-387, 1995.

39. Chez RA: Woman battering, *Am J Obstet Gynecol* 158(1):1-4, 1988.

9 GENITAL TRAUMA

Jenifer Markowitz

Sexual violence often occurs concurrently with physical assaults in domestic violence incidents. According to findings from the National Violence Against Women Survey, an estimated 322,230 intimate partner rapes were committed against women in the United States in the 12 months preceding the survey. This amounts to 3.2 intimate partner rapes per 1000.[1] A survey of men from the same publication found that 0.3% of men reported being raped by an intimate partner at some point in their lifetime ($n = 8000$). There are a number of physical health problems that may arise as a result of sexual abuse. Studies identify multiple health issues for women who have experienced sexual violence, which include gynecologic issues such as vaginal bleeding, urinary tract infections, sexually transmitted infections, and pelvic pain and nongynecologic issues such as hypertension, obesity, and high cholesterol.[2-4] This includes an increased risk for HIV infection.[5] There is evidence that women who experience sexual abuse with or without concurrent physical abuse are more likely to experience these complaints than women who experience physical abuse alone.[2] However, even in the presence of routine clinical screening for domestic violence, questions regarding sexual violence are frequently left unasked.

With this in mind, it is essential that clinicians routinely ask about sexual violence and document signs and symptoms of injuries resulting from forcible sexual contact and direct trauma in both male and female patients (Figure 9-1). A complete rape examination, including an evidence collection kit, should be conducted on any patient who reports forcible sexual contact and is agreeable to the medico-legal examination. These patients should be referred to the closest Sexual Assault Nurse Examiner (SANE) program or emergency department for immediate care if the assault has occurred within 120 hours (depending on the state). After the allotted time, if the patient has not been examined since the assault occurred or if the patient refuses the rape kit, a complete examination is still encouraged, including the following components:

1. Sexually transmitted infection risk evaluation and prophylactic treatment if appropriate
2. Pregnancy evaluation and emergency contraception if appropriate or desired
3. Evaluation, treatment, and documentation of all injuries[6]

There is evidence that documentation of moderate to severe injury increases the likelihood that criminal charges are filed,[7] although lack of genital injury does not negate the seriousness or the impact of the sexual violence.

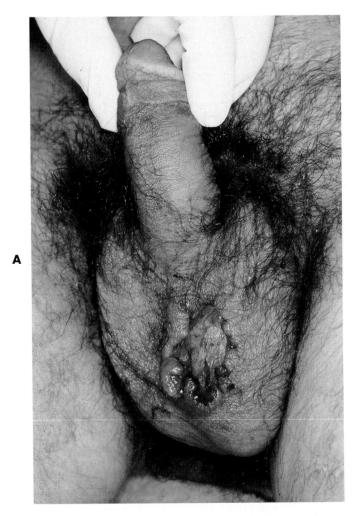

A

FIGURE 9-1   **A,** Scrotal tear. *(Courtesy Dr. David Effron, MetroHealth Medical Center, Cleveland, Ohio.)*

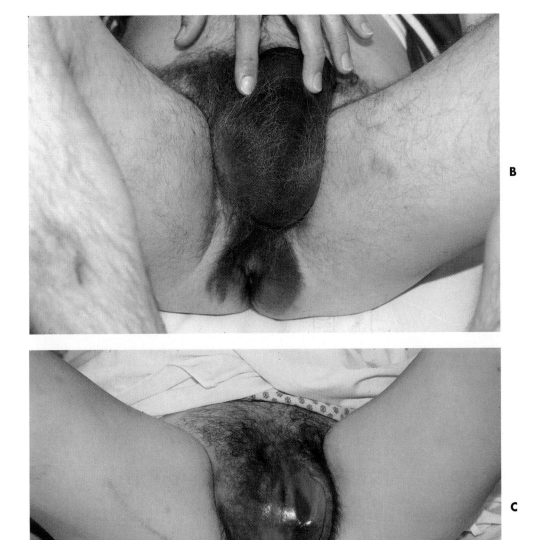

B

C

FIGURE 9-1, cont'd   **B,** Scrotal ecchymosis. *(Courtesy Dr. David Effron, MetroHealth Medical Center, Cleveland, Ohio.)* **C,** Labial hematoma. *(Courtesy Dr. David Effron, MetroHealth Medical Center, Cleveland, Ohio.)*

External genitalia should be carefully examined for abrasions, contusions (Figure 9-2), tears (Figure 9-3), and pattern injuries such as fingernail marks (Figure 9-4) and even bite wounds (Figure 9-5, *A*). The area should be carefully inspected; in female patients this means paying particular attention to areas where injury may be missed, including hymenal tissue, the posterior fourchette, the fossa navicularis, and the labia minora[8] (Figure 9-5, *B*). Slaughter and others found that most injury following forcible sexual contact occurs as a result of a penis or foreign object being inserted or attempted to be inserted into the vagina.[9] Most of the injury secondary to

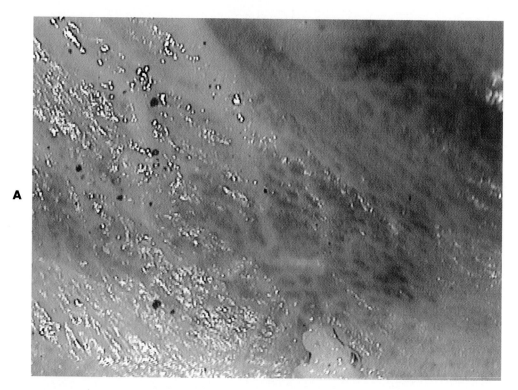

A

FIGURE 9-2   **A,** Posterior fourchette contusion (colposcope ×30). (*Courtesy Dr. Jenifer Markowitz, The DOVE Program, Summa Health System, Akron, Ohio.*)

forcible penetration of the vagina is to one or more of the aforementioned areas[8,10] (Table 9-1). Speculum and/or anoscopic examinations should be conducted per patient history. Injury can be detected using a colposcope for magnification. These injuries can best be captured with a 35-mm or digital camera attached directly to the colposcope. Although there are time constraints for collecting forensic evidence for the rape kit, injury may still be evident at or beyond 72 hours.[9] Therefore the passage of time should not diminish the value of a focused examination for purposes of documenting genital injury.

Text continued on page 147

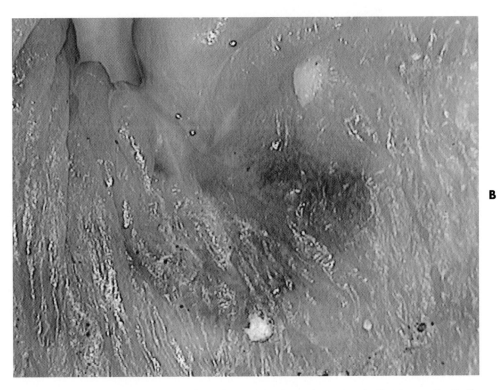

B

FIGURE 9-2, cont'd **B,** Posterior fourchette contusion (colposcope ×15). *(Courtesy Dr. Jenifer Markowitz, The DOVE Program, Summa Health System, Akron, Ohio.)*

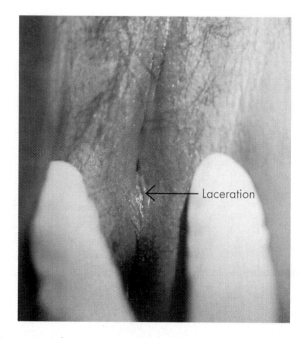

FIGURE 9-3   Laceration of the posterior fourchette. *(From Girardin B and others:* Color atlas of sexual assault, *St Louis, 1997, Mosby.)*

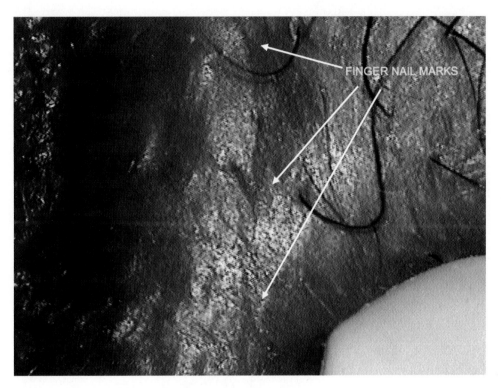

FINGER NAIL MARKS

FIGURE 9-4 Indentations from fingernails *(arrow)* in the labia majora (colposcope ×15). *(Courtesy The DOVE Program, Summa Health System, Akron, Ohio.)*

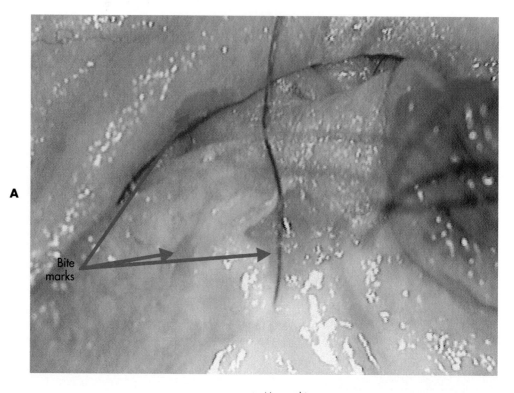

Bite marks

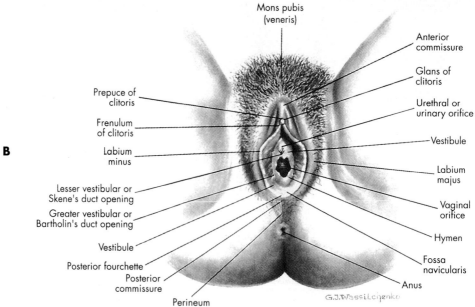

Mons pubis
(veneris)

Anterior
commissure

Glans of
clitoris

Prepuce of
clitoris

Urethral or
urinary orifice

Frenulum
of clitoris

Vestibule

Labium
minus

Labium
majus

Lesser vestibular or
Skene's duct opening

Vaginal
orifice

Greater vestibular or
Bartholin's duct opening

Hymen

Vestibule

Fossa
navicularis

Posterior fourchette

Posterior
commissure

Anus

G.J.Wassilchenko

Perineum

FIGURE 9-5   **A,** Bite marks around the clitoris (colposcope ×30). **B,** Anatomical sites in the external female genitalia. *(A, Courtesy The DOVE Program, Summa Health System, Akron, Ohio. B, From Lowdermilk, DL, Perry, SE, Bobak, IM:* Maternity and women's health care, *ed. 6, St Louis, 1997, Mosby.)*

Table 9-1	*Sites and Types of Genital Injury in Penile Vaginal Penetration*	
SITE	INCIDENCE OF INJURY (%)	TYPES OF INJURY
Posterior fourchette	70	Laceration, abrasion
Labia minora	53	Abrasion, ecchymosis
Hymen	29	Ecchymosis, laceration
Fossa navicularis	25	Laceration, abrasion
Cervix	13	Ecchymosis
Vagina	11	Laceration, ecchymosis
Perineum	11	Laceration, abrasion
Periurethral	9	Ecchymosis
Labia majora	7	Redness, abrasion

From Slaughter L, Brown CRV: Cervical findings in rape victims, *Am J Obstet Gynecol* 164:528, 1991; Slaughter L: Personal communication, December, 1996.

Injury to the female external genitalia may also result from generalized blunt or penetrating trauma incurred during the course of the physical assault. Like other types of injuries, these should also be carefully documented and photographed.

Male patients should be examined carefully, as well, with particular attention to the perineum and perianal areas. It is important to note that injuries surrounding the anus are easily missed, so significant retraction is necessary to adequately visualize the entire area (Box 9-1, Figure 9-6). Any visible injury, regardless of severity should be noted in the written documentation, labeled on a corresponding body map, and photographed. This includes contusions, abrasions, erythema, and swelling. Particular care should be taken to document the mechanism of injury. Although punching and kicking are certainly common, thrown objects are frequently the weapon of choice in partner assaults and their potential for serious harm should not be discounted.[11]

Box 9-1	*Significant Nonspecific Perianal Findings*

FINDINGS PROBABLY RELATED TO NONCONSENSUAL SEXUAL CONTACT	PERIANAL FINDINGS
Distorted, irregular anal folds	Perianal skin tags
	Hyperpigmentation
Immediate (within 30 seconds) dilation ≥20 mm of the anus with no stool palpable or visible within rectal ampulla	Flat or thick anal folds at the 6 o'clock and 12 o'clock positions
	Diastasis ani—smooth area of no folds at the 6 o'clock and 12 o'clock positions
Flaccid rectal tone for first 12 to 48 hours postassault, resulting from damage to external sphincter	Anal fissures
Fixed opening of anus	Anal dilation or opening of the external and internal anal sphincters as a result of feces in rectal ampulla
Rectal sphincter spasm	
Erythema and edema of the perianal tissue with pain and bleeding	Erythema
	Venous congestion causing local or diffuse discoloration
Perianal scar associated with an asymmetry in the shape of the anus when it is closed	Tightening or relaxing of anus when buttocks are spread
Perianal lacerations extending beyond the external anal sphincter	Pain on defecation
	Cellulitis
Semen retrieved from the anal canal	Hemorrhoids

Modified from Adams JA, Knudson S: Genital findings in adolescent girls referred for suspected sexual abuse, *Arch Pediatr Adolesc Med* 150:850, 1996.

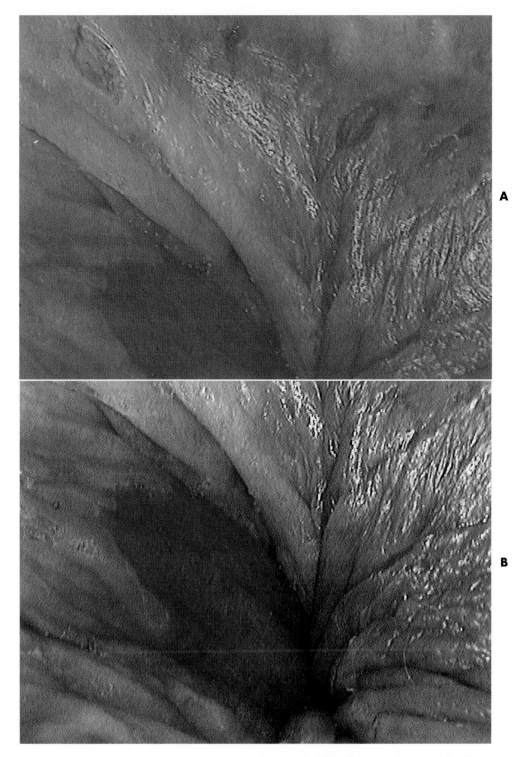

FIGURE 9-6　**A,** Anal laceration (colposcope ×15). **B,** Anal laceration and perianal lacerations following anal-digital penetration (colposcope ×15). *(A, Courtesy The DOVE Program, Summa Health System, Akron, Ohio. B, Courtesy Valorie Prulhiere, RN, BSN, FNE, SANE-A, The DOVE Program, Summa Health System, Akron, Ohio.)*

Of the medically significant external genital injuries seen in men by emergency department physicians, the most common is the traumatic sudden flexion of the penis, otherwise known as the "fractured penis." This injury requires surgical intervention and will present with tenderness, ecchymosis, and swelling of the shaft of the penis.[12]

Injuries to the scrotum and testicles are also seen following both blunt and penetrating trauma. Clinicians should have a high index of suspicion when patients present with scrotal pain and swelling and should not rule out the possibility of trauma-induced testicular torsion as a plausible diagnosis.[13] Seng and Moissinac,[13] in their review of the literature, reported incidence rates of traumatic testicular torsion between 4% and 12%. Immediate investigation is warranted in such events, with appropriate urology or surgery consultation.

Penetrating wounds to the external genitalia, such as impalements and gunshot wounds, will also require immediate surgical consultation (Figure 9-7). Although these wounds can be psychologically, as well as physically traumatic, Brandes and others[14] found that gunshot wounds to the external genitalia, particularly singular gunshot wounds, predominantly resulted in injury to proximal soft tissue and responded well to conservative management.

It is important to note that sexual abuse in the context of domestic violence includes more than just forcible sexual contact. It also includes acts meant to humiliate or degrade, such as forcing a person to watch her partner have sex with other partners. It may also include acts that can result in loss of access to the health care system such as being denied access to birth control or STI treatment.[15] Clinicians must be explicit in their questions regarding sexual violence when screening patients in battering relationships.

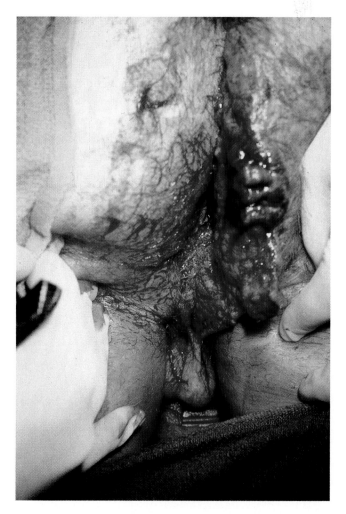

FIGURE 9-7   Impalement injury. *(Courtesy S. Scott Polsky.)*

SUMMARY

Sexual violence is one component of domestic violence. Because approximately 1 in 5 individuals who are victims of physical violence are also victims of sexual violence, clinicians must screen all patients who disclose intimate partner violence. Clinicians must also remember that beyond forcible sexual contact, blunt and penetrating trauma can result in injuries to the external genitalia. Male as well as female patients should be carefully screened for such injuries and care taken to anticipate the potentially emergent conditions that can result from them. As with other types of domestic violence–related injury, consultation with and referral to specialties such as gynecology, urology, and surgery can make treatment of genital injuries more successful, with fewer physical and psychological sequelae.

REFERENCES

1. Tjadenn P, Thoennes N: *Full report of the prevalence, incidence and consequences of intimate partner violence,* Washington, DC, 2000, National Institute of Justice and Centers for Disease Control and Prevention.
2. Cambell J and others: Intimate partner violence and physical health consequences, *Arch Intern Med* 162:1157-1163, 2002.
3. Cloutier S, Martin SL, Poole C: Sexual assault among North Carolina women: prevalence and health risk factors, *J Epidemiol Community Health* 56(4):265-271, 2002.
4. Eby KK and others: Health effects of experiences of sexual violence for women with abusive partners, *Health Care Women Int* 16(6):563-576, 1995.
5. Wyatt GE and others: Does a history of trauma contribute to HIV risk for women of color? Implications for prevention and policy, *Am J Public Health* 92(4):660-665, 2002.
6. Groleau GA, Jackson MC: Forensic examination of victims and perpetrators of sexual assault. In Olshaker JS, Jackson MC, Smock WS, eds: *Forensic emergency medicine,* Philadelphia, 2001, Lippincott Williams & Wilkins.
7. McGregor MJ and others: Examination for sexual assault: Is the documentation of physical injury associated with the laying of charges? *Can Med Assoc J* 160(11):1565-1569, 1999.
8. Girardin BW and others: *Color atlas of sexual assault,* St Louis, 1997, Mosby.
9. Slaughter L and others: Patterns of genital injury in female sexual assault victims, *Am J Obstet Gynecol* 176(3):609-616, 1997.
10. Biggs M and others: Genital injuries following sexual assault of women with and without prior sexual intercourse experience, *Can Med Assoc J* 159(1):33-37, 1998.
11. Markowitz JR, Bunnell J: Unpublished data, The DOVE Program Summa Health System, Akron, Ohio, 2002.
12. Dreitlein DA, Suner S, Basler J: Genitourinary trauma, *Em Med Clin North Am* 19(3):569-590, 2001.
13. Seng YJ, Moissinac K: Trauma induced testicular torsion: A reminder for the unwary, *J Accidental Emerg Med* 17(5):381-382, 2000.
14. Brandes SB and others: External gunshot wounds: a ten-year experience with fifty-six cases, *J Trauma* 39(2):266-271, 1995.
15. Salfer PR, Taliaferro E: *The physician's guide to domestic violence,* Volcano, Calif, 1995, Volcano Press.

10 MUSCULOSKELETAL INJURIES

Lori Sieboldt Lowery • Douglas J. Lowery • Scott D. Weiner

Musculoskeletal injuries sustained as the result of domestic violence often share common presentations. The clinician should attempt to educate himself or herself in pattern recognition to help identify the offending object and therefore more readily identify abuse. For example, patients who are struck with a direct blow from either a fist or wielded object often have a specific injury location. The defensive posture causes injuries to the ulnar aspect of the forearm, and the person sustains the so-called nightstick pattern injury (Figure 10-1). Isolated transverse ulnar fractures are generally not caused by falls. In healthy adults who are not

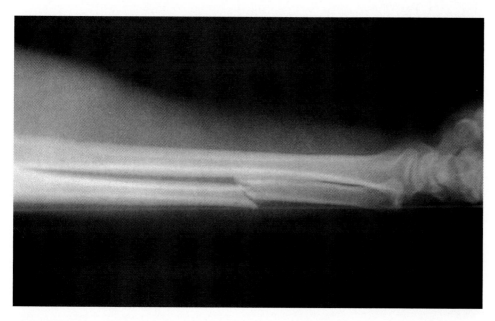

FIGURE 10-1 Radiograph of nightstick fracture. *(Courtesy Scott Weiner, MD, Department of Orthopedic Surgery, Summa Health System, Akron, Ohio.)*

involved with high-energy trauma such as motor vehicle collisions, bilateral wrist injuries may indicate a forceful fall down stairs or being violently thrown to the ground. Orbital blowout fractures, potential bite marks, cigarette burns, and concentrated axial injuries, such as multiple chest or abdomen injuries, should raise suspicion that domestic violence is the underlying cause of the injury. Gunshot wounds may be the result of domestic violence, as may other types of penetrating injuries (Figure 10-2). The orthopedic elements of abuse are varied and sometimes occult. In this regard, consultation with an orthopedic surgeon may help ascertain whether the stated cause or pattern of injury may be the result of domestic violence.

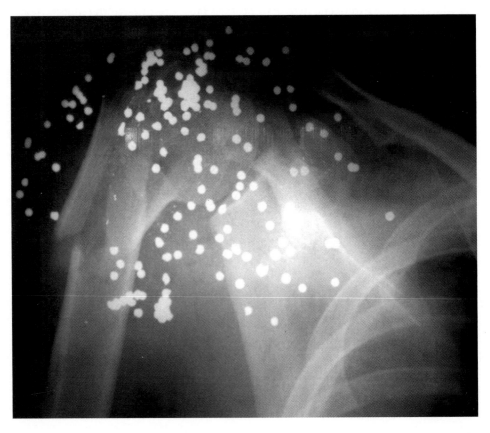

FIGURE 10-2 Radiograph of multiple pellets in the shoulder. *(Courtesy Scott Weiner, MD, Department of Orthopedic Surgery, Summa Health System, Akron, Ohio.)*

PHYSICAL EXAMINATION

It is imperative to do a complete physical examination of any patient suspected as a victim of abuse, to assess for musculoskeletal injuries. It is necessary to disrobe the patient fully to ensure that all surfaces are visually inspected for evidence of trauma. Because many of the areas that indicate abuse are centrally located, concentration on only the injured extremity may jeopardize the acquisition of vital clues to the underlying abuse etiology. As with any trauma, a cursory palpation of all axial and appendicular structures is warranted. Palpation should include full spine examination for point tenderness and step-off, which could be the result of a direct blow. Range of motion of all joints may also demonstrate occult injuries inconsistent with the original complaint.

Any suspicious area should be thoroughly examined as above, and obtaining plain radiographs should be considered. Interpreting the radiograph includes determining whether the stated mechanism of injury is consistent with the pattern of fracture or dislocation. Blunt force trauma secondary to impacts and sudden deceleration generally deform the bone in a bending manner. This produces a characteristic transverse or butterfly pattern (Figure 10-3). Rotational injuries cause long oblique or spiral fractures (Figure 10-4). A skeletal survey is useful in adults as well as in children in cases in which abuse is suspected (Box 10-1). According to the American Academy of Pediatrics, a skeletal survey should include both axial and appendicular radiographs. The extremity views should include anterior-posterior (AP) views of bilateral arms, forearms, hands, thighs, lower legs, and feet. Axial radiographs should include AP and lateral views of the trunk and skull.[1]

A bone scan may be particularly helpful as an adjuvant diagnostic tool in suspected child abuse to demonstrate occult injuries.[2] It may identify multiple fractures in various stages of healing. Suspicious injuries in elders are not always secondary to abuse. Often those with severe osteopenia may have pathologic fracture secondary to metabolic or metastatic processes. A skeletal survey may identify these etiologies and prevent inappropriate accusation. Spine injuries may require computed tomography (CT) or magnetic resonant imaging (MRI) but only after appropriate plain radiographs are obtained. Consultation with an orthopedic surgeon may help determine the most appropriate diagnostic study for a suspected injury.

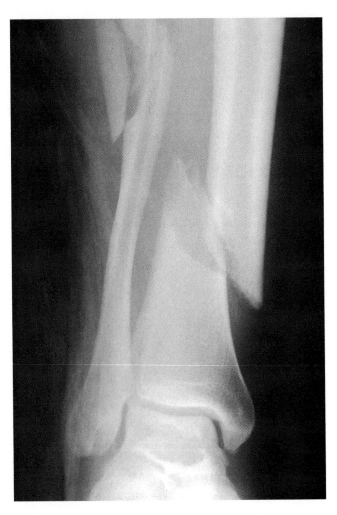

FIGURE 10-3   Radiograph of butterfly pattern fracture. *(Courtesy Scott Weiner, MD, Department of Orthopedic Surgery, Summa Health System, Akron, Ohio.)*

APPENDICULAR SKELETON
- Arms (AP)
- Forearms (AP)
- Hands (AP)
- Thighs (AP)
- Lower legs (AP)
- Feet (PA or AP)

AXIAL SKELETON
- Skull (frontal and lateral)
- Thorax (AP and lateral)
- Abdomen, lumbosacral spine, and bony pelvis (AP)
- Lumbar spine (lateral)
- Cervical spine (AP and lateral)

AP, Anterior-posterior, *PA*, posterior-anterior.
(Data from American College of Radiology: ACR standards for skeletal surveys in children, Reston, Va, 2001, American College of Radiology.)

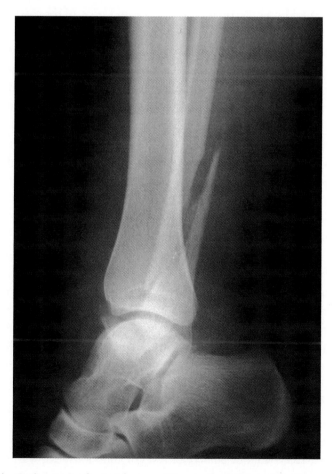

FIGURE 10-4   Radiograph of spiral fracture. *(Courtesy Scott Weiner, MD, Department of Orthopedic Surgery, Summa Health System, Akron, Ohio.)*

INJURY TYPES

Soft tissue trauma encompasses many potential types of injury. Ligamentous sprains and strains of the wrist and ankle are common complaints in the emergency department. Usually isolated twisting-related episodes or specific falls cause these injuries. A pregnant woman though, who presents with bilateral wrist injuries, should prompt the clinician to do a more detailed history and examination, which may uncover other injuries. For example, a common radiocarpal or distal radioulnar joint sprain secondary to simple twisting generally does not demonstrate ecchymosis. Bruising may indicate an inconsistency between the patient's story and physical examination that should be investigated. Contusions about the wrists and ankles in elders are one specific indication of abuse. This is often secondary to being tied down to either a bed or chair. Other suspicious lesions include contusions to the abdomen, breast, chest, or medial aspect of the legs and arms.[3] Most impacts with objects caused by falls occur to extensor surfaces on the upper or lower extremities. Clusters of axial contusions are highly suspicious for abuse.[4] This is especially true for those at-risk populations as discussed above. Patients must be thoroughly examined, including the breasts, abdomen, and back of those who are pregnant. If suspicion or complaint dictates, clinicians must investigate the perineum for trauma.

Fractures in the healthy adult population usually follow a commonly seen pattern. Routine mechanisms and presentations include clavicle fractures resulting from a direct blow to the shoulder or, less commonly, a fall onto an outstretched hand (Figures 10-5 and 10-6). Impacted proximal humerus fractures are often seen in elders, as are unilateral comminuted distal radius fractures, because of the osteoporotic nature of the involved bone. Figures 10-7 and 10-8 are two radiographs of different proximal humerus fractures typical in the elderly population. Uncommon findings should raise concerns in an at-risk population. For example, a distal radius fracture in a young adult (Figure 10-9) is more suspicious because this requires a much higher level of energy. The previously mentioned nightstick fracture is almost always the result of direct trauma to the defensively postured extremity. Multiple rib fractures after a reportedly low-energy fall are also uncommon. In the lower extremity, spiral tibial fractures in a healthy adult may also be a source of skepticism. In children, the malleable nature of immature bone as well as open growth plates helps facilitate identification of suspicious fracture patterns. For example, corner or "bucket handle" fractures, in which the junction of the metaphysis and the epiphysis show a small avulsion in children, have an extremely high correlation with abuse in children.

Spinal injuries are generally related to high-energy impacts such as falls from height or motor vehicle collisions. Some other etiologies known to be associated with spinal trauma include sporting events such as football, wrestling, and track and field (Figure 10-10).

Babies and toddlers often are predisposed to injury secondary to a large head-to-body ratio combined with ligamentous laxity. A direct blow to the neck in an adult may cause ligamentous injury, which may then require flexion and extension spine series, or may demonstrate spinous process fracture (Figure 10-11). Findings that may indicate head or neck trauma, such as contusion, abrasion, laceration, or change of level of consciousness, warrant cervical spine examination and radiographs. As with all spinal pathology, once an injury is discovered

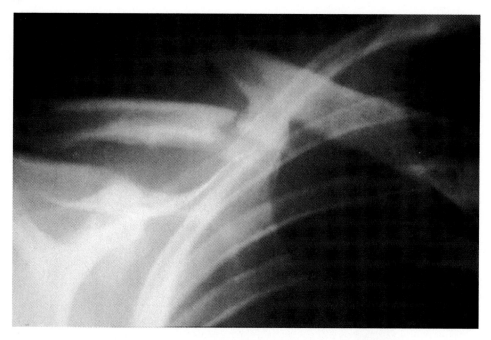

FIGURE 10-5   Radiograph of a clavicle fracture. *(Courtesy Dr. David Effron, MetroHealth Medical Center, Cleveland, Ohio.)*

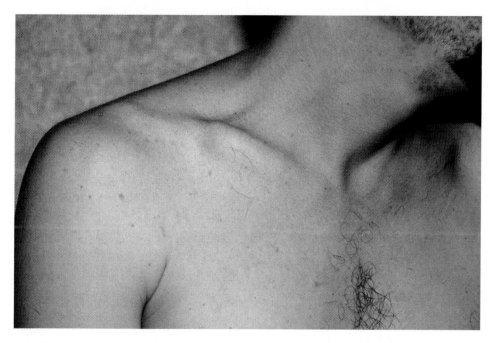

FIGURE 10-6   Clavicle fracture. *(Courtesy Dr. David Effron, MetroHealth Medical Center, Cleveland, Ohio.)*

detailed examination of the entire spine is mandatory. A complete neurologic examination should be undertaken and documented in any case of suspected central nervous system injury. Dislocations in the adult spine would be uncommon from direct blows. Falls down stairs, striking the head against an object during a fall, or severe head or neck trauma generally is required to cause this type of injury in a healthy adult (Figure 10-12). The same is not necessarily true for children or elders.

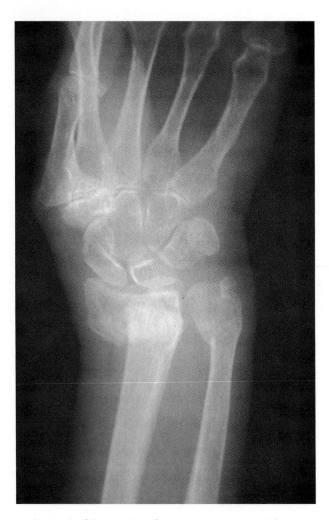

FIGURE 10-7   Radiograph of distal radius fracture typical in the elderly population. *(Courtesy Scott Weiner, MD, Department of Orthopedic Surgery, Summa Health System, Akron, Ohio.)*

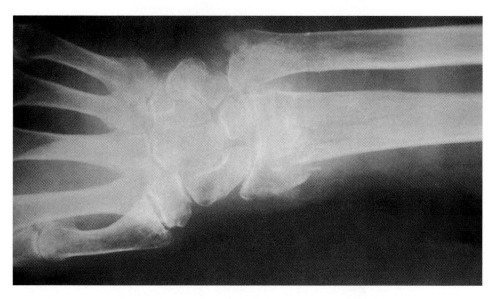

FIGURE 10-8   Radiograph of distal radius fracture typical in the elderly population. *(Courtesy Scott Weiner, MD, Department of Orthopedic Surgery, Summa Health System, Akron, Ohio.)*

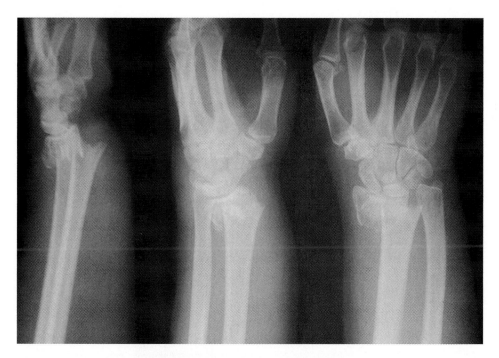

FIGURE 10-9   Radiograph of young person, high-energy wrist fracture in three views. *(Courtesy Scott Weiner, MD, Department of Orthopedic Surgery, Summa Health System, Akron, Ohio.)*

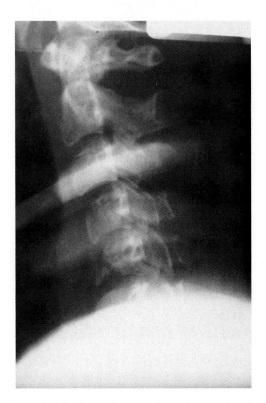

FIGURE 10-10   Radiograph of a burst fracture, C5. *(Courtesy Dr. David Effron, MetroHealth Medical Center, Cleveland, Ohio.)*

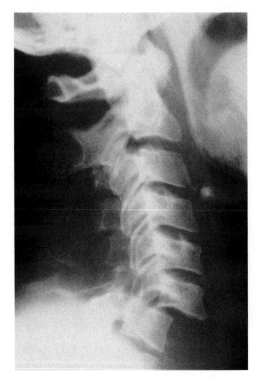

FIGURE 10-11   Radiograph of bilateral facet dislocation, C6 to C7 and clay shovelers. *(Courtesy Dr. David Effron, MetroHealth Medical Center, Cleveland, Ohio.)*

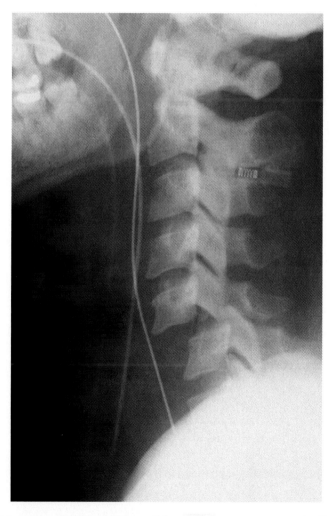

FIGURE 10-12 C5 to C6 bilateral facet dislocation. *(Courtesy Dr. David Effron, MetroHealth Medical Center, Cleveland, Ohio.)*

SUMMARY

Treatment of musculoskeletal injuries caused by abuse should follow the standard of care in the community. Documentation of each specific injury may be crucial for the patient and clinician if legal action should ensue. In fact, if a battered patient is treated by a clinician who does not inquire into possible domestic violence, that clinician may be held liable for subsequent injuries sustained by returning the victim to her original environment.[2] All members of the treatment team involved in the care of the patient should be made aware of the potential circumstances surrounding the incident so that proper documentation as well as follow-up can be provided appropriately. For those patients who may face obstacles in accessing care, many clinicians will accommodate them with more flexible office hours. Because many of the victims have children, the entire family may need to receive care once the underlying cause is identified. Clinicians of all disciplines, including specialists, may contribute their expertise in caring for the family. Knowledge of the mandatory guidelines/action plan in the emergency department may help facilitate these efforts.

REFERENCES

1. American Academy of Pediatrics Section on Radiology: Diagnostic imaging of child abuse, *Pediatrics* 87:262-264, 1991.
2. Zillmer DA: Domestic violence: the role of the orthopaedic surgeon in identification and treatment, *J Am Acad Orthop Surg* 8(2):91-96, 2000.
3. Guth AA, Pachter HL: Domestic violence and the trauma surgeon, *Am J Surg* 179:134-140, 2000.
4. Burge SK: Violence against women, *Primary Care Clin Office Pract* 24(1):67-81, 1997.

11 PATIENT POPULATIONS AND SPECIAL CONSIDERATIONS

Jenifer Markowitz • Valorie K. Prulhiere

As with so many public health issues, intimate partner violence must be examined in the context of race, class, age, gender, culture, and sexuality. Although it transcends all of these, it is also affected by each, and it is important for the clinician to understand that there is not one blanket approach for dealing with domestic violence in the general patient population. Screening, treatment, and referral must be approached with these concepts in mind to maximize their efficacy. This chapter seeks to introduce or reunite clinicians with the special issues of a variety of patient populations and provide resources for further information.

LESBIAN, GAY, TRANSGENDERED, AND BISEXUAL (LGTB) PATIENTS

According to the Family Violence Prevention Fund, available studies suggest that there is no difference between the rates of domestic violence in the heterosexual and homosexual communities. Furthermore, unlike in the heterosexual community, where the vast majority of domestic violence victims are women, in the homosexual community, victims are as likely to be male as female.[1] Clinicians need to be cognizant of this and pay special attention to screening and referral techniques, which will be inclusive of all patients, regardless of sexual orientation[1]:

- Do not assume the gender of the assailant.
- Do not assume that no children are involved because the couple in question is a same-sex partnership.
- Do not assume that a patient's willingness to disclose sexual orientation to you means that patient wants other community agencies and law enforcement personnel to have that information as well.
- Do not assume that sexual violence is the exclusive province of heterosexual relationships.
- Do not assume that a same-sex relationship could be any less potentially lethal than a heterosexual relationship

Keep in mind that issues such as homophobia, lack of family support, and denial in the gay and lesbian community about the incidence and prevalence of domestic violence may make it harder for patients to disclose battering. It may also make finding support services more difficult. In addition, the legal system may be less likely to take the violence seriously or even to categorize it as domestic violence.[1] These issues need to be considered for the safety and well-being of LGTB patients.

As with any victim of domestic violence, screening of LGTB patients should be direct and nonjudgmental and should be implemented consistently. A lesser approach would be unethical and potentially dangerous. Refer to Additional Resources listed at the end of this chapter for further information regarding domestic violence resources in the LGTB community and for LGTB-specific information for health care providers.

PATIENTS WITH DISABILITIES

According to the Center for Research on Women With Disabilities, approximately 55% of women with disabilities reported a history of emotional, physical, or sexual abuse, similar to rates for women without disabilities. However, women with disabilities were more likely to remain in abusive relationships for longer periods than women without disabilities.[2] The National Center for Injury Prevention and Control, in a review of research on sexual violence against people with disabilities, report that most data indicate that people with disabilities are at higher risk for sexual violence than people without disabilities.[3] Clinicians must be aware that victims who are disabled often have fewer economic resources and frequently are limited by community resources ill equipped to handle special-needs clientele. The disabled victim may also experience a type of abuse other populations would not normally have to cope with: caregiver abuse. Caregiver abuse includes physical, emotional, and sexual abuse. However, it also includes the withholding of crucial medication, equipment, or transportation necessary for activities of daily living.[4] Fortunately, the extent of violence against individuals with disabilities has become more widely recognized; in 2000, the reauthorization of the Violence Against Women Act strengthened supports for women with disabilities.[5]

Clues to domestic violence in the patient's medical history or examination are no different from those in the general population. All suspected or confirmed violence must be charted accordingly, and appropriate referrals must be made. Safety must be the priority. Although domestic violence should always be handled by a team approach, it is the authors' experience that it is especially important in cases of victims with disabilities to involve other disciplines to help establish realistic and adequate safety plans, community referrals, and follow-up. Communication among medical disciplines also should occur so that the patient with multiple health care providers can receive the best possible care with an eye toward continuing safety and effective treatment options in the context of potentially ongoing violence in the home. Clinicians should familiarize themselves with area resources for the disabled and inquire about the ability of local shelters to cope with both the physically and mentally disabled. Clinicians should also be aware of shelter accessibility for the physically disabled, as well as shelter policies regarding alcohol and drug intoxication so that a plan can be implemented for those victims who battle addiction. For more information on domestic violence resources for the disabled, refer to Additional Resources at the end of this chapter.

CULTURE AND DOMESTIC VIOLENCE

Domestic violence crosses all cultural boundaries. This does not mean, however, that all cultural groups react to domestic violence in the same manner, either from an individual or a community perspective. Although some may tout "recipes" for treating particular ethnic or religious groups, such approaches are fundamentally flawed because they simply perpetuate community stereotypes. Therefore the clinician should consider each patient's care individually, taking into account various cultural and racial issues but avoiding assumptions based on either. There are a host of national resources specific to various cultures; some of these are dedicated solely to the issue of domestic violence. For recommended readings, Internet sites, and national organizations, refer to Additional Resources at the end of this chapter.

CHILDREN WHO WITNESS VIOLENCE

Children can be physically injured in the course of domestic violence incidents or during coexisting child-abuse events. Studies report a 30% to 60% overlap between domestic violence and child abuse in the same families.[6] Christian and others[7] found that unlike child abuse injuries, however, injuries sustained during domestic violence incidents rarely displayed identifiable patterns. Furthermore, these injuries usually were noted to be related to domestic violence incidents only because the children presented with the history of family violence or in some cases because of clinician investigation into family history of violence. Injuries directly related to domestic violence incidents may be missed altogether if screening for such violence is not done routinely.

Injury that occurs from witnessing domestic violence is less simple to identify and can be as insidious as physical abuse.[8] There are no reliable national prevalence data for children who have witnessed domestic violence, in part because of wide variations in study definitions.[9] However, factors have been identified that may influence the degree to which witnessing such violence affects children. These include the following[10]:

- Co-occurrence of abuse and witnessing domestic violence
- Characteristics of the child, including age and gender
- Length of time since the violent event
- Parent–child relationships, including child perceptions of these relationships
- External family support

In 2000, the U.S. Department of Justice released a report from the National Summit on Children Exposed to Violence. *Safe From the Start* outlines eight operating principles to address children's exposure to violence[11]:

- Work together.
- Begin earlier.
- Think developmentally.
- *Make mothers safe to keep children safe* (italics are the author's).
- Enforce the law.
- Make adequate resources available.
- Work from a sound knowledge base.
- Create a culture of nonviolence.

Although these do not wholly pertain to health care providers, they do provide a foundation from which clinicians can approach the problem, particularly in a multidisciplinary fashion. Refer to Additional Resources at the end of this chapter for information about *Safe From the Start* and other resources for children who have witnessed domestic violence.

ELDERLY VICTIMS

The National Elder Abuse Incident Study estimated that in 1996 almost half a million elders were victims of abuse and/or neglect in domestic settings.[12] This does not include victims living in institutional settings. Elderly victims of domestic violence may or may not be included in general elder abuse statistics, because the two are not necessarily interchangeable. As with other types of violence, identification and documentation are essential. Every patient should be screened, regardless of chief complaint and regardless of gender. The National Committee for the Prevention of Elder Abuse suggests several ways in which clinicians can play a role in early intervention. These include the following[13]:

- Identification of somatic signs and symptoms of abuse
- Evaluation of the plausibility of explanations given for common injuries and conditions
- Provision of expert testimony
- Assessment of cognitive status and health factors that affect it
- Treatment of injuries or health problems arising from abuse

Many resources are available to assist clinicians in caring for elderly victims. Refer to Additional Resources at the end of this chapter for recommended readings, Internet sites, and national organizations.

SUMMARY

Domestic violence transcends age, race, gender, culture, class, and sexuality. There is no typical profile of the domestic violence victim. However, patients cannot be treated in a vacuum; screening must be universal, and treatment and discharge plans must be created on an individual basis. There is no one answer for the patient living with violence. Clinicians can best help their patients by being aware of community resources which meet the needs of a variety of patient populations and by familiarizing themselves with the breadth of literature on this topic.

REFERENCES

1. Family Violence Prevention Fund: *Responding to domestic violence in lesbian, gay, transgender and bisexual communities,* San Francisco, 1999, The Fund.
2. Center for Research on Women with Disabilities (www.bcm.tmc.edu/crowd/abuse_women/ABUGUIDE.htm accessed 3/14/02): *Guidelines for physicians on the abuse of women with disabilities,* Houston, 1999, The Center.
3. National Center for Injury Prevention and Control (http://www.cdc.gov/ncipc/factsheets/disabvi.htm accessed 3/27/02): *Sexual violence against people with disabilities,* Atlanta, Centers for Disease Control and Prevention.
4. National Center for the Dissemination of Disability Research (www.ncddr.org/rr/women/priorities.html#footnote_1 accessed 11/2/02): *Priorities for future research: results of BPA's Delphi Survey of disabled women,* Oakland, Calif, 1997, Berkeley Planning Associates.

5. Office of Victims of Crime: *First response to victims of crime who have a disability,* Washington, DC, 2002, U.S. Department of Justice.

6. National Clearinghouse on Child Abuse and Neglect Information (http://www.calib.com/nccanch/pubs/otherpubs/ harmsway.cfm accessed 11/02/02): *In harm's way: domestic violence and child maltreatment,* Washington, DC, US Department of Health and Human Services.

7. Christian CW and others: Pediatric injury resulting from family violence, *Pediatrics* 99(2):E8.

8. Margolin G: Effects of domestic violence on children. In Trickett, PK, Schellenbach, CJ, eds: *Violence against children in the family and the community.* Washington, DC, 1998, American Psychological Association.

9. Fantuzzo JW, Mohr WK: Prevalence and effects of child exposure to domestic violence, *Future Child Domestic Violence Child* 9(3):21-32, 1999.

10. Edleson J: *Problems associated with children's witnessing of domestic violence,* 1997, Violence Against Women On-Line Resources (www.vaw.umn.edu/VAWnet/witness.htm).

11. Office of Juvenile Justice and Delinquency Prevention: *Safe from the start: taking action on children exposed to violence,* Washington, DC, 2000, US Department of Justice.

12. Administration on Aging: *The national elder abuse incident study (executive summary),* Washington, DC, 1998, US Department of Health and Human Services.

13. National Committee for the Prevention of Elder Abuse: *Health and medical* (www.preventelderabuse.org accessed 4/3/02).

ADDITIONAL RESOURCES

GAY, LESBIAN, BISEXUAL, AND TRANSGENDERED

Publications

Girshick LB: *Women to women sexual violence,* Boston, 2002, Northeastern University Press.

Renzetti CM, Miley CH, eds: *Violence in gay and lesbian domestic partnerships,* Binghampton, NY, 1996, Harrington Park Press.

Lundy SE, Leventhal B, eds: *Same-sex domestic violence: strategies for change,* Thousand Oaks, Calif, 1999, Sage Press.

Organizations

Gay Men's Domestic Violence Project
955 Massachusetts Avenue
PMB 131
Boston, MA 02139
1-800-832-1901 (crisis line)
(617) 354-6056 (office)

Gay and Lesbian Medical Association
459 Fulton Street
Suite 107
San Francisco, CA 94102
(415) 255-4547 (office)
http://www.glma.org

Lambda Gay and Lesbian Community Services
PO Box 31321
El Paso, TX 79931-0321
(915) 329-GAYS (office)
http://www.lambda.org

PATIENTS WITH DISABILITIES
Publications

Salber PR, Taliaferro E: *The physician's guide to domestic violence,* Volcano, Calif, 1995, Volcano Press.

Institute on Community Integration, The College of Education and Human Development, University of Minnesota: Violence and women with developmental or other disabilities, *Impact* 13(3:)Feature Issue, 2000. (http://ici.umn.edu)

Website

CAVNET (Communities Against Violence Network)*
http://www.cavnet2.org

Guidelines for Physicians on the Abuse of Women With Disabilities
http://www.bcm.tmc.edu/crowd/abuse_women/ABUGUIDE.htm

National Women's Health Information Center
http://www.4woman.gov/wwd/abuse.htm

CULTURE AND DOMESTIC VIOLENCE
Publications

Bohn DK: Lifetime and current abuse, pregnancy risks and outcomes among Native American women, *J Healthcare Poor Underserved* 13(2):184-198, 2002

Jasinski JL: Physical violence among Anglo, African-American and Hispanic couples: ethnic differences in persistence and cessation, *Violence Victim* 16(5):479-490, 2001.

National Clearinghouse on Family Violence: *Family violence in aboriginal communities: an aboriginal perspective,* Ottawa, Ontario, 1996, Health Canada.
http://www.hc-sc.gc.ca/hppb/familyviolence/html/1abor.html

National Clearinghouse on Family Violence: *A resource guide on family violence issues for aboriginal communities,* Ottawa, Ontario, 1994, Health Canada.
http://www.hc-sc.gc.ca/hppb/familyviolence/html/fvabor/1fvabor.html

McNutt L, and others: Partner violence and medical encounters: African-American women's perspectives, *Am J Prev Med* 19(4):264-269, 2000.

McDonnell KA, Abdulla SE, Project AWARE: *Report on the study of abused Asian women,* Washington, DC, 2002, The Asian/Pacific Islander Domestic Violence Resource Project (http://www.dvrp.org).

*This site is an excellent resource for a variety of violence-related issues.

Peek-Asa C and others: Severity of intimate partner abuse indicators as perceived by women in Mexico and the United States, *Women's Health* 35(2-3):181-192, 2002.

Short LM, Rodriguez R: Testing an intimate partner violence assessment icon form with battered migrant and seasonal farmworker women, *Women's Health* 35(2-3):181-192, 2002.

Video

Center for the Prevention of Sexual and Domestic Violence: *Broken vows: religious perspectives on domestic violence,* Seattle, 1994, The Center (www.cpsdv.org).

Center for the Prevention of Sexual and Domestic Violence: *To save a life: ending domestic violence in Jewish families,* Seattle, 1997, The Center (www.cpsdv.org).

Websites

Asian and Pacific Islander Health Forum
http://www.apiahf.org

Institute on Domestic Violence in the African-American Community
http://www.dvinstitute.org

Jewish Women International
http://www.jewishwomen.org

Migrant Clinician's Network Domestic Violence Services
http://www.migrantclinician.org/education/famvio.html

National Latin Alliance for the Elimination of Domestic Violence
http://www.dvalianza.org

National Network on Behalf of Battered Immigrant Women
http://endabuse.org/programs/immigrant/

Native American Domestic Violence Information
http://www.letswrap.com/nadvinfo/

CHILDREN WHO WITNESS VIOLENCE
Publications

Culross PL: Health care system response to children exposed to domestic violence, *Future Child* 9(3 Winter), 1999), The David and Lucille Packard Foundation.
http://www.futureofchildren.org/

Fantuzzo JW, Mohr WK: Prevalence and effects of child exposure to domestic violence, *Future Child* 9(3 Winter), 1999, The David and Lucille Packard Foundation.
http://www.futureofchildren.org/

Edelson J: *Problems associated with children's witnessing of domestic violence,* 1999, Violence Against Women Online Resources (VAWnet). http://www.vaw.umn.edu/Vawnet/witness.htm

Office of Juvenile Justice and Delinquency Prevention: *Safe from the start: taking action on children exposed to violence,* Washington, DC, 2000, US Department of Justice.

Websites

Children's Defense Fund
http://www.childrensdefense.org

Family Violence Department of the National Council of Juvenile and Family Court Judges
http://www.dvlawsearch.com/

National Center for Children Exposed to Domestic Violence
http://www.nccev.org

National Clearinghouse on Child Abuse and Neglect Information
http://www.calib.com/nccanch

Our Children Our Future Charitable Foundation
http://www.ocof.org

ELDERLY VICTIMS

Publications

US Department of Health and Human Services: Administration on Aging, *The national elder abuse incidence study: final report,* Washington, DC, 1998, US DHHS. http://www.aoa.gov/abuse/report/default.htm.

Kapp MB: Criminal and civil liability of physicians for institutional elder abuse and neglect, *J Am Med Direct Assoc* 2(4):155-159, 2001.

American Medical Association: *Diagnostic and treatment guidelines on elder abuse and neglect,* Chicago, The Association. http://www.ama-assn.org

Websites

National Center on Elder Abuse
http://www.elderabusecenter.org/

National Committee for the Prevention of Elder Abuse: Health and Medical Professionals
http://www.preventelderabuse.org/professionals/medical.htm

United States Department of Justice: Elder Justice
http://www.usdoj.gov/elderjustice.htm

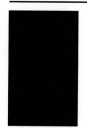

APPENDICES

APPENDIX A
PROFESSIONAL ORGANIZATIONS

American Academy of Family Physicians
11400 Tomahawk Creek Parkway
Leawood, KS 66221-2672
Phone: (913) 906-6000
E-mail: fp@aafp.org
www.aafp.org

American Academy of Nurse Practitioners
P.O. Box 12846
Austin, TX 78711
Phone: (512) 442-4262
Fax: (512) 442-6469
www.aanp.org

American Academy of Orthopedic Surgeons
6300 N. River Road
Rosemont, IL 60018-4262
Phone: (800) 346-AAOS
Fax: (847) 823-8125
Fax on demand: (800) 999-2939
www.aaos.org

American Academy of Pediatrics
141 Northwest Point Boulevard
Elk Grove Village, IL 60007-1098
Phone: (847) 434-4000
Fax: (847) 434-8000
www.aap.org

American Academy of Physician Assistants
950 N. Washington Street
Alexandria, VA 22314-1552
Phone: (703) 836-2272
Fax: (703) 684-1924
E-mail: aapa@aapa.org
www.aapa.org

American Association of Occupational Health Nurses
50 Lenox Pointe
Atlanta, GA 30324-3176
Phone: (404) 262-1162
www.aaohn.org

American Association of Oral and Maxillofacial Surgeons
9700 W. Bryn Mawr Avenue
Rosemont, IL 60018-6200
Phone: (847) 678-6200
www.aaoms.org

The American College of Emergency Physicians
1125 Executive Circle
Irving, TX 75038-2522
Phone: (800) 798-1822 or (972) 550-0911
Fax: 972-580-2816
www.acep.org

American College of Nurse-Midwives
818 Connecticut Avenue N.W.
Suite 900
Washington, DC 20006
Phone: (202) 728-9860 (front desk)
Fax: (202) 728-9897
Fax on demand: (202) 728-9898
E-mail: info@acnm.org
www.acnm.org

American College of Nurse Practitioners
2401 Pennsylvania Avenue N.W.
Washington, DC 20037-1718
Phone: (202) 466-4825
www.nurse.org/acnp

American College of Obstetricians
  and Gynecologists
409 12th Street S.W.
P.O. Box 96920
Washington, DC 20090-6920
Phone: (800) 320-0610
Fax: (202) 728-0617
www.acog.org
E-mail: violence@acog.org

American College of Physicians/American
  Society of Internal Medicine
190 North Independence Mall West
Philadelphia, PA 19106-1572
Phone: (800) 338-2746
www.acponline.org

American Dental Association
211 E. Chicago Avenue
Chicago, IL 60611
Phone: (312) 440-2500
Fax: (312) 440-2800
www.ada.org

American Medical Association
515 N. State Street
Chicago, IL 60610
Phone: (312) 464-5000
www.ama-assn.org

American Nurses Association
600 Maryland Avenue S.W.
Suite 100 West
Washington, DC 20024
Phone: (202) 651-7000
Fax: (202) 651-7001
www.ana.org

American Psychiatric Association
1400 K Street N.W.
Washington, DC 20005
Phone: (888) 357-7924
Fax: (202) 682-6850
E-mail: apa@psych.org
www.psych.org

Association of Pediatric Nurse
  Practitioners
20 Brace Road
Suite 200
Cherry Hill, NJ 08034-2633
Phone: (856) 857-9700
Fax: (856) 857-1600
E-mail: info@napnap.org
www.napnap.org

Association of Women's Health, Obstetric
  and Neonatal Nurses (AWHONN)
2000 L Street N.W.
Suite 740
Washington, DC 20036
Phone: (800) 673-8499 (USA)
Phone: (800) 245-0231 (Canada)
Fax: (202) 728-0575
www.awhonn.org

Emergency Nurses Association
915 Lee St.
Des Plaines, IL 60016-6569
Phone: (800) 900-9659
www.ena.org

International Association of Forensic Nurses
East Holly Avenue
Box 56
Pitman, NJ 08071-0056
Phone: (856) 256-2425
Fax: (856) 589-7463
www.forensicnurse.org
E-mail: iafn@ajj.com

National Association of Emergency Medical Technicians
408 Monroe Street
Clinton, MS 39056-4210
Phone: (800) 35-NAEMT
Fax: (601) 924-7325
E-mail info@naemt.org
http://www.naemt.org

National Association of Nurse Practitioners in Women's Health
503 Capitol Court N.E.
Suite 300
Washington, DC 20002
Phone: (202) 543-9693
Fax: (202) 543-9858
E-mail: info@npwh.org
www.npwh.org

National Conference of Gerontological Nurse Practitioners
P.O. Box 270101
Fort Collins, CO 80527-0101
Phone: (970) 493-7793
www.ncgnp.org

Office of the Surgeon General
5600 Fishers Lane
Room 18-66
Rockville, MD 20857
www.osophs.dhhs.gov

Society of Thoracic Surgeons
401 N. Michigan Avnue
Chicago, IL 60611-4267
Phone: (312) 321-6803
Fax: (312) 527-6635
E-mail: sts@sba.com
www.sts.org

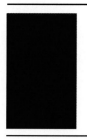

APPENDIX B
SUGGESTED SCREENING QUESTIONS

FRAMING QUESTIONS

➡ Because violence is so common in many people's lives, I've begun to ask all my patients about it.

➡ I'm concerned that your symptoms may have been caused by someone hurting you.

➡ I don't know if this is a problem for you, but many of the women I see as patients are dealing with abusive relationships. Some are too afraid or uncomfortable to bring it up themselves, so I've started asking about it routinely.

➡ Some of the lesbian women and gay men we see here are hurt by their partners. Does your partner ever try to hurt you?

DIRECT VERBAL QUESTIONS

➡ Are you in a relationship with a person who physically hurts or threatens you?

➡ Did someone cause these injuries? Was it your partner/husband?

➡ Has your partner or ex-partner ever hit you or physically hurt you? Has he ever threatened to hurt you or someone close to you?

➡ Do you feel controlled or isolated by your partner?

➡ Do you ever feel afraid of your partner? Do you feel you are in danger? Is it safe for you to go home?

➡ Has your partner ever forced you to have sex when you didn't want to? Has your partner ever refused to practice safe sex?

Modified from forms developed by the Family Violence Prevention Fund and Educational Programs Associates, Inc. *Continued*

FOR HISTORY INTAKE FORMS/
NEW PATIENT QUESTIONNAIRES

OPTION 1

➡ Have you ever been hurt or threatened by your boyfriend/husband/partner?

-OR-

➡ Have you ever been hit, kicked, slapped, pushed, or shoved by your boyfriend/husband/partner?

-OR-

➡ Have you ever been hit, kicked, slapped, pushed, or shoved by your boyfriend/husband/partner during this pregnancy?

-AND-

➡ Have you ever been raped or forced to engage in sexual activity against your will?

OPTION 2

➡ Are you currently or have you ever been in a relationship where you were physically hurt, threatened, or made to feel afraid?

OPTION 3

➡ Have you ever been forced or pressured to have sex when you did not want to?

➡ Have you ever been hit, kicked, slapped, pushed or shoved by your boyfriend/husband/partner?

Modified from forms developed by the Family Violence Prevention Fund and Educational Programs Associates, Inc.

OPTION 4

ABUSE ASSESSMENT SCREEN

1. Have you ever been emotionally or physically abused by your partner or someone important to you?   ❑ Yes   ❑ No
2. Within the last year, have you been hit, slapped, kicked, or otherwise physically hurt by someone?   ❑ Yes   ❑ No

   If Yes, by whom? _____ Total number of times: _____
3. Since you've been pregnant, were you hit, slapped, kicked, or otherwise physically hurt by someone?   ❑ Yes   ❑ No

   If Yes, by whom? _____ Total number of times: _____

Mark the area of injury on a body map.
Score each incident according to the following scale:
1 = Threats of abuse including use of a weapon
2 = Slapping, pushing, no injuries and/or lasting pain
3 = Punching, kicking, bruises, cuts, and/or continuing pain
4 = Beating up, severe contusions, burns, broken bones
5 = Head injury, internal injury, permanent injury
6 = Use of weapon; wound from weapon
If any of the descriptions for the higher number apply, use the higher number.

---

4. Within the last year, has anyone forced you to have sexual activities?
                                         ❑ Yes   ❑ No

   If Yes, by whom? _____ Total number of times: _____
5. Are you afraid of your partner or anyone you listed above?   ❑ Yes   ❑ No

OPTION 5

For use as a rubber stamp or printed on Intake Form:

SCREENING	❑ Yes	❑ No	*or*	**SCREENING**		
❑ DV+	❑ DV−	❑ DV?		❑ DV+	❑ DV−	❑ DV?

(Note: "DV?" means that domestic violence is suspected.)

Modified from forms developed by the Family Violence Prevention Fund and Educational Programs Associates, Inc.   *Continued*

DOMESTIC VIOLENCE SCREENING/DOCUMENTATION FORM

DV Screen
❑ DV+ (Positive)
❑ DV? (Suspected)

Date _____ Patient ID# _____
Patient Name _____
Provider Name _____
Patient Pregnant?   ❑ Yes ❑ No

ASSESS PATIENT SAFETY

❑ Yes ❑ No   Is abuser here now?
❑ Yes ❑ No   Is patient afraid of his/her partner?
❑ Yes ❑ No   Is patient afraid to go home?
❑ Yes ❑ No   Has physical violence increased in severity?
❑ Yes ❑ No   Has partner physically abused children?
❑ Yes ❑ No   Have children witnessed violence in the home?
❑ Yes ❑ No   Threats of homicide?
If Yes, by whom: _____
❑ Yes ❑ No   Threats of suicide?
If Yes, by whom: _____
❑ Yes ❑ No   Is there a gun in the home?
❑ Yes ❑ No   Alcohol or substance abuse?
❑ Yes ❑ No   Was safety plan discussed?

REFERRALS

❑ Hotline number given
❑ Legal referral made
❑ Shelter number given
❑ In-house referral made
Describe: _____
❑ Other referral made
Describe: _____

REPORTING

❑ Law enforcement report made
❑ Child Protective Services report made
❑ Adult Protective Services report made

PHOTOGRAPHS

❑ Yes ❑ No   Consent to be photographed?
❑ Yes ❑ No   Photographs taken?
Attach photographs and consent form.

Developed by the Family Violence Prevention Fund and Educational Programs Associates, Inc.

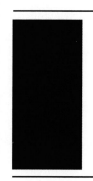

APPENDIX C
RESOURCES FOR INFORMATION ABOUT PATIENT POPULATIONS AND SPECIAL CONSIDERATIONS*

GAY, LESBIAN, BISEXUAL AND TRANSGENDERED

Publications

Annual report on lesbian, gay, bisexual, and transgender domestic violence.
http://www.lambda.org

The Health Resource Center on Domestic Violence, Family Violence Prevention Fund: *Responding to domestic violence in lesbian, gay, transgendered and bisexual communities.*
http://www.endabuse.org

Renzetti CM, Miley CH, editors: *Violence in gay and lesbian domestic partnerships,* Binghampton, NY, 1996, Harrington Park Press.

Lundy SE, Leventhal B, editors: *Same-sex domestic violence: strategies for change,* Thousand Oaks, Calif, 1999, Sage Press.

Organizations
Gay Men's Domestic Violence Project
955 Massachusetts Avenue
PMB 131
Boston, MA 02139
Phone: (800) 832-1901 (crisis line)
Phone: (617) 354-6056 (office)

Gay and Lesbian Medical Association
459 Fulton Street
Suite 107
San Francisco, CA 94102
Phone: (415) 255-4547 (office)
http://www.glma.org

Lambda Gay and Lesbian Community Services
P.O. Box 31321
El Paso, TX 79931-0321
Phone: (915) 329-GAYS (office)
http://www.lambda.org

* Please note this is by no means an exhaustive list of available information. For further information, we recommend searching the Minnesota Center Against Violence and Abuse Electronic Clearinghouse (http://www.mincava.umn.edu), one of the best online resources available for information about violence.

PATIENTS WITH DISABILITIES
Publications
Salber PR, Taliaferro E: *The physician's guide to domestic violence,* Volcano, Calif, 1995, Volcano Press.

National Center for Injury Prevention and Control, Centers for Disease Control and Prevention: *Sexual violence against people with disabilities fact sheet,* Author.
http://www.cdc.gov/ncipc/factsheets/disabvi.htm

Institute on Community Integration, The College of Education and Human Development, University of Minnesota: Violence and women with developmental or other disabilities, *Impact* 13(3:) Feature Issue, 2000.
http://www.ici.umn.edu

Websites
Guidelines for Physicians on the Abuse of Women With Disabilities
http://www.bcm.tmc.edu/crowd/abuse_women/ABUGUIDE.htm

CULTURE AND DOMESTIC VIOLENCE
Publications
National Clearinghouse on Family Violence: *Family violence in aboriginal communities: an aboriginal perspective,* Ottawa, Ontario, 1996, Health Canada.
http://www.hc-sc.gc.ca/hppb/familyviolence/html/1abor.htm

National Clearinghouse on Family Violence: *A resource guide on family violence issues for aboriginal communities,* Ottawa, Ontario, 1994, Health Canada.
http://www.hc-sc.gc.ca/hppb/familyviolence/html/fvabor/1fvabor.html

McNutt L and others: Partner violence and medical encounters: African-American women's perspectives, *Am J Prev Med* 19(4):264-269, 2000.

Project AWARE: *Report on the study of abused Asian women,* The Asian/Pacific Islander Domestic Violence Resource Project.
http://www.dvrp.org

Videos
Center for the Prevention of Sexual and Domestic Violence: *Broken vows: religious perspectives on domestic violence,* Seattle, 1994, The Center.

Websites
Asian and Pacific Islander Health Forum
http://www.apiahf.org

Institute on Domestic Violence in the African-American Community
http://www.dvinstitute.org

Migrant Clinician's Network Domestic Violence Services
http://www.migrantclinician.org/education/famvio.html

National Latin Alliance for the Elimination of Domestic Violence
http://www.dvalianza.org

National Network on Behalf of Battered Immigrant Women
http://endabuse.org/programs/immigrant/

Native American Domestic Violence Information
http://www.letswrap.com/nadvinfo/

CHILDREN WHO WITNESS VIOLENCE

Publications

Culross PL: *Health care system response to children exposed to domestic violence, Future Child* 9(3) (Winter 1999), The David and Lucille Packard Foundation.
http://www.futureofchildren.org

Fantuzzo JW, Mohr WK: *Prevalence and effects of child exposure to domestic violence, Future Child* 9(3) (Winter 1999), The David and Lucille Packard Foundation.
http://www.futureofchildren.org

Edelson J: *Problems associated with children's witnessing of domestic violence,* 1999, Violence Against Women Online Resources (VAWnet).
http://www.vaw.umn.edu/Vawnet/witness.htm

U.S. Department of Justice, Office of Juvenile Justice and Delinquency Prevention: *Safe from the start: taking action on children exposed to violence,* Washington, DC, 2000, Author.

Websites

Children's Defense Fund
http://www.childrensdefense.org

Family Violence Department of the National Council of Juvenile and Family Court Judges
http://www.dvlawsearch.com/

National Center for Children Exposed to Domestic Violence
http://www.nccev.org

National Clearinghouse on Child Abuse and Neglect Information
http://www.calib.com/nccanch

Our Children Our Future Charitable Foundation
http://www.ocof.org

ELDERLY VICTIMS

Publications

U.S. Department of Health and Human Services, Administration on Aging: *The national elder abuse incidence study: final report,* Washington, DC, 1998, Author.
http://www.aoa.gov/abuse/report/default.htm

Kapp MB: Criminal and civil liability of physicians for institutional elder abuse and neglect, *J Am Med Direct Assoc* 2(4):155-159, 2001.

American Medical Association: *Diagnostic and treatment guidelines on elder abuse and neglect,* The Association.
http://www.ama-assn.org

Websites

National Center on Elder Abuse
http://www.elderabusecenter.org

National Committee for the Prevention of Elder Abuse: Health and Medical Professionals
http://www.preventelderabuse.org/professionals/medical.htm

United States Department of Justice: Elder Justice
http://www.usdoj.gov/elderjustice.htm

TEEN DATING VIOLENCE

Publications

Silverman JG and others: Dating violence against adolescent girls and associated substance use, unhealthy weight control, sexual risk behavior, pregnancy, and suicidality, *JAMA* 286(5):572-579, 2001.

National Center for Injury Prevention and Control, Centers for Disease Control and Prevention: *Dating violence fact sheet,* 2000, Author.
http://www.cdc.gov/ncipc/factsheets/datviol.htm

Websites

Break the Cycle: Empowering Youth to End Domestic Violence
http://www.break-the-cycle.org

Love Is Not Abuse (Liz Claiborne Women's Work)
http://www.lizclaiborne.com/loveisnotabuse/default.asp

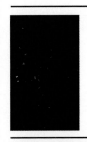

APPENDIX D
STATE REPORTING STATUTES

State Reporting Statutes

STATE (STATUTE)	INJURIES FROM WEAPONS	INJURIES FROM CRIMES	INJURIES FROM DOMESTIC VIOLENCE*
Alabama	No	No	No
Alaska (Statute 08.64.369)	Yes	Yes	No
Arizona (Rev Stat 13-3806)	Yes	Yes	No
Arkansas (Code Ann 12-12-602)	Yes	No	No
California (Pen Code 11172 AB74X19)	Yes	Yes	Yes
Colorado (Rev Stat 12-36-135)	Yes	Yes	Yes
Connecticut (Acts 269)	Yes	No	No
Delaware (Code Ann 24-17-1762)	Yes	No	No
District of Columbia (Ann 2-1361)	Yes	No	No
Florida (Stat Ann 790.24)	Yes	Yes	No
Georgia (Code Ann 31-7-9)	No	Yes	No
Hawaii (Rev Stat 453-14)	Yes	Yes	No
Idaho (Code 39-1390)	Yes	Yes	No
Illinois (Code Ann 20-2630-3)	Yes	Yes	No
Indiana (Code Ann 35-47-1)	Yes	No	No
Iowa (Code Ann 147.111)	Yes	Yes	No
Kansas (Stat 21-4213)	Yes	No	No
Kentucky (Stat Ann 209.020)	No	Yes	Yes
Louisiana (Rev Stat 403.5)	Yes	No	No
Maine (Rev Stat 17A Ch 21.512)	Yes	No	No
Maryland (Ann Code 336, art 27)	Yes	No	No
Massachusetts (Gen Laws 112-12)	Yes	No	No
Michigan (Comp Laws 750.411)	Yes	Yes	No
Minnesota (Stat Ann 626.52)	Yes	No	No
Mississippi (Code Ann 45-9-31; 93-21-1)	Yes	No	Yes
Missouri (Rev Stat 578-350.1)	Yes	Yes	No
Montana (Code Ann 37-2-302)	Yes	No	No
Nebraska (Rev Stat 28-902)	No	Yes	No

*Verified as of March 2001. Please refer to individual state statutes to determine the specific parameters for reporting domestic violence injury. Some states, such as Ohio, do not mandate reporting of *all* domestic violence injuries, only cases in which certain characteristics exist (e.g., disability injury). Other states, such as Colorado, mandate reporting *all* domestic violence injury.
Houry D and others: Violence-inflicted injuries: reporting laws in the fifty states, *Ann Emerg Med,* 39:58, 2002.   *Continued*

State Reporting Statutes—cont'd

STATE (STATUTE)	INJURIES FROM WEAPONS	INJURIES FROM CRIMES	INJURIES FROM DOMESTIC VIOLENCE
Nevada (Rev Stat Ann 629.041)	Yes	No	No
New Hampshire (Rev Stat Ann 631.6)	Yes	Yes	No
New Jersey (Stat Ann 2C: 58-8)	Yes	No	No
New Mexico	No	No	No
New York (Penal Code 265.25)	Yes	No	No
North Carolina (Gen Stat 90-21.20)	Yes	Yes	No
North Dakota (Cent code 43-17-41)	Yes	Yes	No
Ohio (ORC 2921; 2151)	Yes	Yes	Yes
Oklahoma (Stat 2105-846.1)	No	Yes	No
Oregon (Rev Stat 146.750)	Yes	No	No
Pennsylvania (Cons Stat Anns 18-5106)	Yes	Yes	No
Rhode Island (Gen Laws 12-29-9; 11-47-48)	Yes	No	Yes
South Carolina	No	No	No
South Dakota (Codified Laws 23-13-10)	Yes	No	No
Tennessee (Stat 36-3-621; 38-1-101)	Yes	Yes	Voluntary
Texas (Fam Code 91.003, 161.041)	Yes	No	Yes
Utah (Code Ann 26-23a)	Yes	Yes	No
Vermont (Stat Ann 13-4012)	Yes	No	No
Virginia (Code Ann 54.1-2967)	Yes	No	No
Washington	No	No	No
West Virginia (Code Ann 61-2-27)	Yes	No	No
Wisconsin (Stat Ann 146.995)	Yes	Yes	No
Wyoming	No	No	No
Total (including DC) "yes"	42	23	7

*Verified as of March 2001. Please refer to individual state statutes to determine the specific parameters for reporting domestic violence injury. Some states, such as Ohio, do not mandate reporting of *all* domestic violence injuries, only cases in which certain characteristics exist (e.g., disability injury). Other states, such as Colorado, mandate reporting *all* domestic violence injury.

Houry D and others: Violence-inflicted injuries: reporting laws in the fifty states, *Ann Emerg Med,* 39:58, 2002.

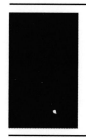

APPENDIX E
COMMUNICATION TOOLS

VAR
Validation, Assessment, Referral
A MODEL FOR SUPPORTING VICTIMS OF DOMESTIC VIOLENCE

Women are more inclined to discuss domestic violence
if they perceive that you are caring and easy to talk to, and if you offer follow-up.
A woman needs to know that the person who asked the question is prepared to deal with her answer.

VALIDATION

What not to say

➤ "The two of you need to go to a marriage counselor, so you can learn better ways to communicate."
Domestic abuse is not a "couples" issue, where each of them is partly responsible for the abuse.

➤ What did you do to make him so angry?"
She already believes (because he has told her so) that she is provoking his attacks. She needs confirmation that his violence is not her fault.

➤ "Here's what you have to do next."
It is not your job to save or rescue her. You can't fix something that may have gone on for years.

➤ What's the matter with you? Don't you care about your children? You can't stay with him a minute longer!
She's in a complex situation, and leaving is not as easy as it seems. A woman is in greatest danger in the six months after she gets out than at any other time.
No woman ever "just leaves" an abuser—she escapes.

What to say

➤ *Statements that communicate your concern.*
"I'm worried about you."
"I'm here to listen, if you want to talk."
"I can give you a referral if you want to talk to someone else about this."

➤ *Statements that clarify her situation.*
"What he's doing to you is wrong."
"It doesn't matter what you did; nobody has the right to treat you this way."

➤ *Statements that acknowledge the complexity of her situation.*
"I know it's hard for you to see the right thing to do. But, in my experience, abuse doesn't go away on its own."
"This isn't an easy decision for you to make. I know you want to do what's best for your children, and that you're worried about finances. There's a lot for you to think about."

➤ *Statements that provide her with tools.*
"I'd like to give you the phone number of the shelter here in town."
"Our city has a victim advocate who works as a volunteer to help you learn about your legal rights. Would you like someone to call her for you?"

➤ "You may not be ready to leave yet. But when you are ready, I will support you. And there are also people in the community who can help."

ABUSERS USE A WIDE RANGE OF TACTICS TO ACHIEVE CONTROL

Control Through Criticism
- ❑ My partner makes me feel like I never do anything right. Nothing is ever good enough.
- ❑ My partner never gives me positive support. Even his compliments are backhanded: "This is the first good dinner you've cooked in months."
- ❑ Whenever we're out with family and friends, I'm on pins and needles because I expect to be humiliated about something I've done.

Control Through Neglect
- ❑ My partner expects me to drop my activities whenever and wherever he wants my attention, but he never pays that kind of attention to me.
- ❑ My partner shows up unannounced whenever he wants to, or fails to show up when he said he would, so I can never make any plans or commitments to others.
- ❑ When I try to express my opinion, he doesn't respond, walks away, or makes fun of me.

Control Through Threats
- ❑ When we have an argument, my partner tells me that I am "acting like a crazy woman." He says that if I don't shape up, he'll have me committed to a mental institution.
- ❑ My partner says that if I ever leave him, he'll kill himself and I'll be responsible.
- ❑ My partner threatens to tell social services that I'm an unfit mother if I don't do what he wants.

Control Through Misrepresentation
- ❑ My partner says cruel things and then says I'm too sensitive and can't take a joke.
- ❑ My partner says he can help me fix my character defects. Then he makes lists of what's wrong with me and tells me I need to see a psychiatrist.
- ❑ When I try to have a serious talk, my partner says, "There you go again, being hysterical. Calm down." He treats me like I'm upset when I'm not.

Control Through Decision Making
- ❑ My partner does the grocery shopping because he says I'm too stupid to pick the right food.
- ❑ My partner picks out my clothes because he says he has better taste than I do, and he knows what outfits suit me.
- ❑ I don't have any say in where we live, how we spend our leisure time, or who we see socially.

Control Through Jealousy
- ❑ When we are at a party and I talk to a man, I always have to keep an eye out for the expression on my partner's face.
- ❑ My partner makes me change my outfit if I put on something that he thinks makes me look like a tramp.
- ❑ If I come home late, my partner accuses me being out with a man or having an affair.

Control Through Money
- ❑ My partner won't give me a household allowance, so whenever I need money I have to ask him for it.
- ❑ My partner gives me everything I want, but he always reminds me that I could never live so well without him.
- ❑ I keep trying to get information about our financial situation, but my partner says I have enough to do without being bothered by money.

Control Through Blame
- ❑ My partner says that he can't stay clean and sober because I don't keep the house clean and the kids quiet.
- ❑ My partner says he wouldn't go after other women if I were thinner, prettier, smarter, and sexier.
- ❑ My partner says he's always good-natured with other people, so that proves it must be what I do that makes him lose control of himself.

Control Through Isolation
- ❑ Whenever I want to go out, my partner always picks that time to start a fight.
- ❑ My partner says I never give him enough time and energy. He accuses me of caring more about my friends and family than about him.
- ❑ If I make a new friend at work or in the neighborhood, my partner always finds something wrong with her.

Control Through Sex
- ❑ My partner forces me to dress in ways he thinks are sexy. It makes me uncomfortable to be out like that in public.
- ❑ My partner pressures me to have sex in ways that make me uncomfortable. When I object, he says I'm frigid.
- ❑ My partner forces me to have sex against my will. He says it isn't rape, because we are a couple and he has the right to take what he wants from me.

Control Through Physical Intimidation
- ❑ My partner blocks the door so I can't leave during a fight.
- ❑ He stands very close to me and clenches his fists. Once, he pinned me to the wall and punched his fist against the wall close to my head.
- ❑ My partner drives recklessly whenever he is angry with me, and it scares me to death.

Control Through Physical Violence
- ❑ My partner throws things at me.
- ❑ My partner beats my head against the wall.
- ❑ My partner chokes me, kicks me, shoves me, bites me, pushes me, and punches me.
- ❑ My partner attacks me with a weapon.

© 2000 Elaine Weiss, EdD.

Dr. Weiss is the author of *Surviving Domestic Violence: Voices of Women Who Broke Free* and *The Family and Friend's Guide to Domestic Violence,* Volcano Press.

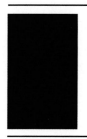

APPENDIX F
SAMPLE FORENSIC
EXAMINATION DOCUMENTATION

CONSENT FOR FORENSIC EXAM, TREATMENT AND RELEASE OF EVIDENCE AND INFORMATION

CONSENT FOR TREATMENT

    I recognize my need for medical care and consent to hospital and forensic services as ordered by the attending physician and his/her designees, including anesthesia, laboratory procedures, medical or surgical treatment, forensic examination and collection of evidence, x-ray examinations, blood/blood products or other medical services rendered under the general and specific orders of the physician and/or designee.

CONSENT FOR RELEASE OF EVIDENCE

    I have received a detailed description of the forensic examination and disclosure process and understand that I may withdraw my consent to any or all parts of the forensic examination at any time except to the extent that action has already been taken having relied upon this authorization.

    (Check one of the two boxes below)

    ❏ *I authorize* the release of evidence, clothing and photograph documentation of injuries to a law enforcement agency for use only in the investigation and prosecution of this crime.

    ❏ *I do not authorize* the release of evidence, clothing or photograph documentation of injuries to a law enforcement agency for use in the investigation and prosecution of this crime. I understand that I may choose to authorize the release of the evidence at a later time by notifying Summa's Forensic Services Department and signing a written release of the evidence.

_____   _____

Patient or Authorized Representative   Date

REVISED 3/2002

Modified from forms developed by The DOVE Program, Summa Health System, Akron, OH.   *Continued*

DOVE PROGRAM
SUMMIT COUNTY
DOMESTIC VIOLENCE NURSE EXAMINER PROGRAM

Social Security # (Case #): _____   Date: _____   DVNE Arrival Time: _____

Name: _____
                    Last Name   First Name   Middle Initial

Age: _____   Date of Birth: _____   Gender: ❑ Male ❑ Female   Race: _____

Address: _____   Home Phone Number: (   ) _____

City: _____   State: _____   Zip: _____   County: _____

DVNE _____

Law Enforcement Officer: _____   Law Enforcement Officer I.D. No.: _____

Report No.: _____   Department: _____

Others Accompanying Victim: _____

Mode of Arrival: Self   Family Member   Friend   Police   EMS   Other

Referring Clinician/Agency: _____

Vital Signs: (If warranted)

Admission:		P		R		BP	
Discharge:		P		R		BP	

Medical History:

Allergies: _____

Last Tetanus: _____

Current Medications: _____

Chronic Medical Conditions
(headache, chronic pain, mental health issues): _____

Acute Illnesses: _____

Past Surgeries: _____

LMP: _____

Are you pregnant or is it possible you might be pregnant at this time: ❑ Yes   ❑ No   ❑ Unsure

If yes, who provides your prenatal care? _____

REVISED 3/2002

Modified from forms developed by The DOVE Program, Summa Health System, Akron, OH.

SUMMIT COUNTY DOMESTIC VIOLENCE NURSE EXAMINER PROGRAM
HISTORY OF ASSAULT

Date of the Assault: _____ Time of the Assault: _____

Location (where the assault occured): _____

Victim's relationship to offender: _____

Name of offender: _____ Address of offender: _____

Are you a previous victim of domestic abuse: ❑ Yes   ❑ No

If yes, list the dates: _____

Previous injuries incurred: _____

Previous medical treatment: ❑ Yes   ❑ No

Previous photographs taken: ❑ Yes   ❑ No

Previous TPO/CPO(s):   ❑ Yes   ❑ No

TYPE OF ABUSE (CURRENT INCIDENT)

PHYSICAL   **PSYCHOLOGICAL**   **SEXUAL**

Check if the following has occurred: **Anatomy involved**

Punching, slapping or kicking   _____

Hit by a thrown item   _____

Grabbing   _____

Hit by an object (please identify)   _____

Physical restraints   _____

Biting   _____

Strangled   _____

Burns   _____

Loss of consciousness   _____

Other   _____

Threats of harm?   ❑ Yes   ❑ No   Type (verbal, weapon, etc.) _____

_____

Children in the home?   ❑ Yes   ❑ No   Ages of children: _____

Children also abused?   ❑ Yes   ❑ No

If yes, have children received medical treatment?   ❑ Yes   ❑ No

If yes, where did they receive treatment? _____

REVISED 3/2002

Modified from forms developed by The DOVE Program, Summa Health System, Akron, OH.   *Continued*

PHYSICAL EXAMINATION

Date of Examination: _____   **Time of Examination:** _____

General Appearance (include condition of clothing): _____

_____

_____

Emotional Status (objective observation): _____

Body Surface (locate and describe injuries, draw the findings on the attached body map)

Mouth/Face: _____

_____

Head/Neck: _____

_____

Back/Buttocks: _____

_____

Chest/Breast: _____

_____

Abdomen: _____

_____

Upper Extremities: _____

_____

Lower Extremities: _____

_____

External Genitalia: _____

_____

Present During the Exam: _____

REVISED 3/2002

Modified from forms developed by The DOVE Program, Summa Health System, Akron, OH.

Narrative History (as described by victim)

REVISED 3/2002

Modified from forms developed by The DOVE Program, Summa Health System, Akron, OH.

Continued

PHOTOGRAPHS

TYPE

☐ 35 mm

☐ Polaroids

☐ Digital

Number of photographs taken: _____   Photographs taken by: _____

Record injuries and findings on diagrams: erythema, abrasions, bruise (detail shape), contusions, induration, lacerations, fractures, bites, burns, stains and foreign materials on the body.

Right   Posterior   Anterior   Left

REVISED 3/2002

Modified from forms developed by The DOVE Program, Summa Health System, Akron, OH.

DIGITAL PHOTOGRAPHY (if applicable)

Client Safety Assessment

1. Is patient afraid to return home? ☐ Yes ☐ No

2. Is there an increase in severity or frequency of abuse? ☐ Yes ☐ No

3. Is there a firearm in the home? ☐ Yes ☐ No

4. If there are child witnesses, have they been referred to the CWWV Program? ☐ Yes ☐ No

Discharge plans: (please specify where patient will go once he/she leaves The DOVE Program)_____

_____

_____

_____

_____

_____

_____

Referrals made: (please list)

1) _____

2) _____

3) _____

4) _____

5) _____

6) _____

REVISED 3/2002

Modified from forms developed by The DOVE Program, Summa Health System, Akron, OH. *Continued*

SPECIMEN COLLECTION AND RECEIPT OF EVIDENCE
(if applicable)

ITEMS COLLECTED

Clothing (list articles):   Yes   No   Not Applicable

Number of Bags: _____

Debris (describe type and location):   Yes   No   Not Applicable

PHOTOGRAPHS	Yes	No	N/A	OTHER:		Yes	No	N/A
FINGERNAIL SCRAPINGS	Yes	No	N/A	OTHER:		Yes	No	N/A
HEAD HAIR (pulled)	Yes	No	N/A	OTHER:		Yes	No	N/A
ORAL SWABS (2)	Yes	No	N/A					
ORAL SMEARS	Yes	No	N/A					
DRIED SALIVA (standard)	Yes	No	N/A					
BITE MARK SWAB	Yes	No	N/A					

Examiner's Name: _____

I have received the above items:

Officer's Name (Printed): _____

Officer's Signature: _____   **I.D. No.:** _____

Law Enforcement Agency: _____

Evidence Released By: _____   **Date:** _____   **Time:** _____

Modified from forms developed by The DOVE Program, Summa Health System, Akron, OH.

STRANGULATION FORM

History
Please mark all that apply:

- ❏ LOC
- ❏ Difficulty/pain with swallowing
- ❏ Loss of voice or voice changes
- ❏ Drooling
- ❏ Breathing difficulties

- ❏ Involuntary urination/defecation during event
- ❏ Loss of memory
- ❏ Coughing
- ❏ Persistent throat pain

Physical Exam
Please mark all that apply:

- ❏ Swelling/edema
- ❏ Coughing
- ❏ Drooling
- ❏ Loss of voice or voice changes
- ❏ Combativeness/irritability/restlessness
- ❏ Uncontrollable shaking
- ❏ Hyperventilation
- ❏ Dyspnea/apnea

Right   Left

Method of Strangulation

- ❏ One hand   ❏ Two hands   ❏ Ligature   ❏ Approached from front
- ❏ Approached from behind   ❏ Other (please describe) _____

Number of times patient was strangled during incident: _____

Number of different methods used for strangulation during incident: _____

Checklist

- ❏ Assess for emergent situation
- ❏ Photograph patient demonstrating (but not physically touching) the strangulation event
- ❏ Examine scalp, eyelids, conjunctiva, chin, jaw, shoulders, and chest
- ❏ Home-going instructions for patient

Modified from forms developed by The DOVE Program, Summa Health System, Akron, OH.

INDEX

Page numbers followed by b indicate box. Page numbers followed by f indicate figure.
Page numbers followed by t indicate table

American College of Emergency Physicians,
176
domestic violence clinical findings, 6, 7b
American College of Nurse-Midwives, 177
American College of Nurse Practitioners, 177
American College of Obstetrics and
Gynecology (ACOG), 177
violence screening protocols, 8
American College of Physicians/American
Society of Internal Medicine, 177
American College of Surgeons
recommendations for severe injuries, 125
statement on domestic violence, 57
American Dental Association, 177
American Dental Association, violence
screening protocols, 8
American Medical Association, 177
American Nurses Association, 177
violence screening protocols, 8
American Psychiatric Nurse, 177
AMPLE history, 60
Anal abrasion, 149f
Anatomic and physiologic changes,
pregnancy and, 132, 134
Anatomic sites in external female genitalia,
146f
Aneurysm, dissecting of, 116f
Anterior chamber, blood in, 82
Aorta, ruptured, 107, 116-117
AP and lateral views, 159b
Arms, defensive laceration of, 55f
Arterial blood gases (ABGs), chest trauma
and, 118
Aspiration risk, in injured pregnant women,
132
Assessment
of blunt abdominal trauma, 123-124
Campbell's Danger Assessment, 9, 10b
danger, 10b
disability, 59
of domestic violence, 3, 12b
fetal, injuries and, 135

Association of Pediatric Nurse Practitioners,
177
Association of Women's Health, Obstetric
and Neonatal Nurses (AWHONN), 177
*ATLS. See Advanced Trauma Life Support
(ATLS)*
Attendance outcomes, work and, 134
AVPU, in assessing level of consciousness, 59
Avulsion, 17t
AWHONN. *See* Association of Women's
Health, Obstetric and Neonatal Nurses
(AWHONN)

B
Ballistics, 63, 65
Battered women, number seeking care,
134
Battering relationship, staying with, 5b, 6b
Battle sign, 83
BB shot, 70
chest multiple gunshot fragments, 71f
Beck's Triad, 116
Bilateral and AP views, 159b
Bilateral facet dislocation
C5-C6, 165f
C6-C7 and clay shovelers, 164f
Bisexual patients, domestic violence and,
167-168
Bite(s), 39
around the clitoris, 149f
impression, 41f
mark on an adult, 42f
tongue, 99f
Bleeding (subcutaneous), ecchymosis and,
123
Blood pressure, pregnancy and, 132
Breathing, 59
chest trauma and, 121
Bruising
contusions, 17, 17t, 20
from heavy workboot, 39f
Buckshot, 70